NATIONAL
MARITIME MUSEUM
GREENWICH

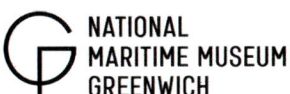

SPOTLIGHT SERIES

Sea Sick

Lime Juice and Scurvy

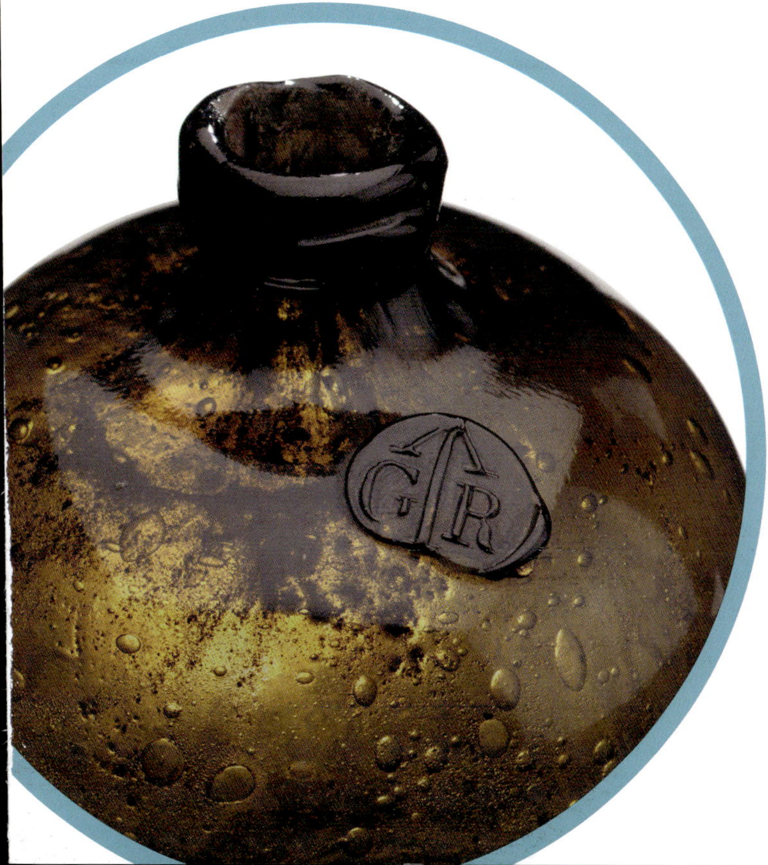

Lucy Dale

A
TREATISE
ON THE
SCURVY.

IN THREE PARTS,

CONTAINING

An Inquiry into the Nature, Cauſes, and Cure, of that Diſeaſe.

Together with

A Critical and Chronological View of what has been publiſhed on the Subject.

Contents

Chapter 1
What Is Scurvy? 4

Chapter 2
A Disease of the Sea 16

Chapter 3
The Search for a Cure 38

Chapter 4
The Discovery of Vitamin C 74

Further Reading 91
Acknowledgements 92
Picture Credits 95

Chapter 1
What Is Scurvy?

The provision of 'lime juice' to Royal Naval ships became official practice in 1795. The lime juice bottle pictured here (figs 1 and 2) can be dated more specifically by its stamp 'GR', meaning it was issued during the reign of George III (r. 1760–1820). Although referred to as a lime juice bottle, it's worth noting that we cannot be certain if the bottle contained lime or rather lemon juice, since the names were used interchangeably at the time. What we do know is that bottles like these were supplied for one reason only – to combat a disease which led to the deaths of an estimated two million seafarers between 1500 and 1800.

In 1589, Richard Hakluyt's (about 1552–1616) *Principall Navigations* makes reference to 'skurvie', marking one of the first uses of the term in an English publication. Of course, other countries had their own names for an illness that recognised no national boundaries. In Dutch, the disease came to be known as *schverbaujckm*, in Danish as *scorbuck*, and in a Latinised term coined by a Dutch physician as *scorbutus*. Nowadays, we know the disease, caused by a lack of vitamin C, simply as scurvy.

The symptoms of scurvy are varied and complex. Observers across the centuries noted that it appeared more as a collection of distinct diseases than a singular illness, making it difficult to diagnose. Thomas Trotter (1760–1832), physician and author of *Observations on the Scurvy with a Review of the Theories Lately Advanced on that Disease* provided a vivid account of its manifestation. Victims lost their strength, their limbs ached, spots formed on the skin, the legs swelled 'with a slight discolouration' and ulcerated, while, in the most infamous of symptoms, the gums blackened and rotted, swelling over teeth which eventually fell out. Trotter noted that as the disease advanced:

> […] the respiration is oppressed on the slightest exertion, with a proneness to faint in an erect posture […] it is not

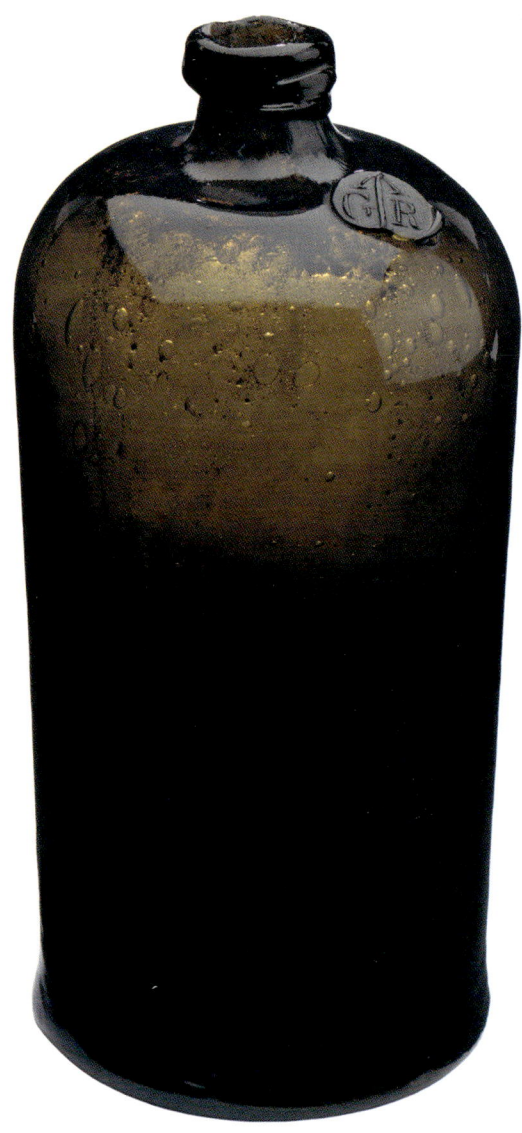

FIG. 1
Lime juice bottle,
late eighteenth century,
glass, 268mm, ZBA7971

FIG. 2
Detail of the seal
of Lime juice Bottle

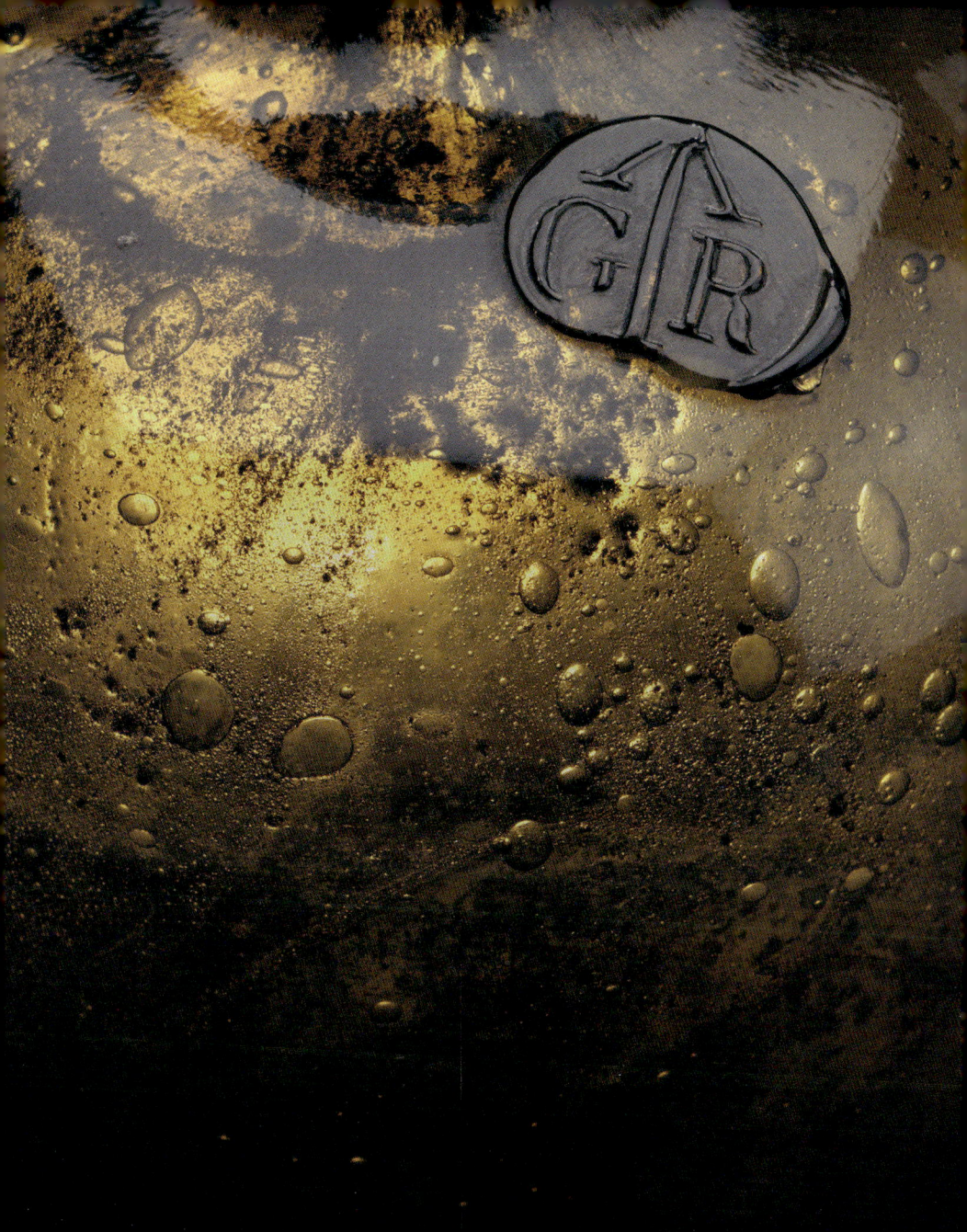

FIG. 3
Plate 10 from Samuel Taylor Coleridge's *Rime of the Ancient Mariner*, Gustave Doré, 1866, engraving, 330 × 482mm, published by Josef Müller, Munich, 1925

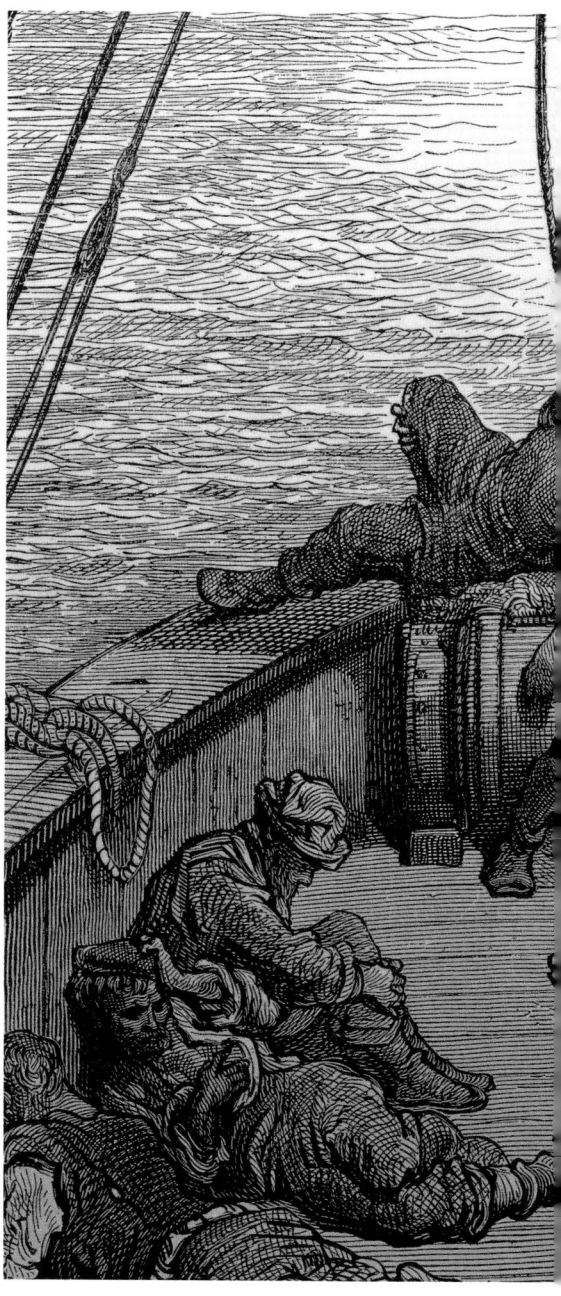

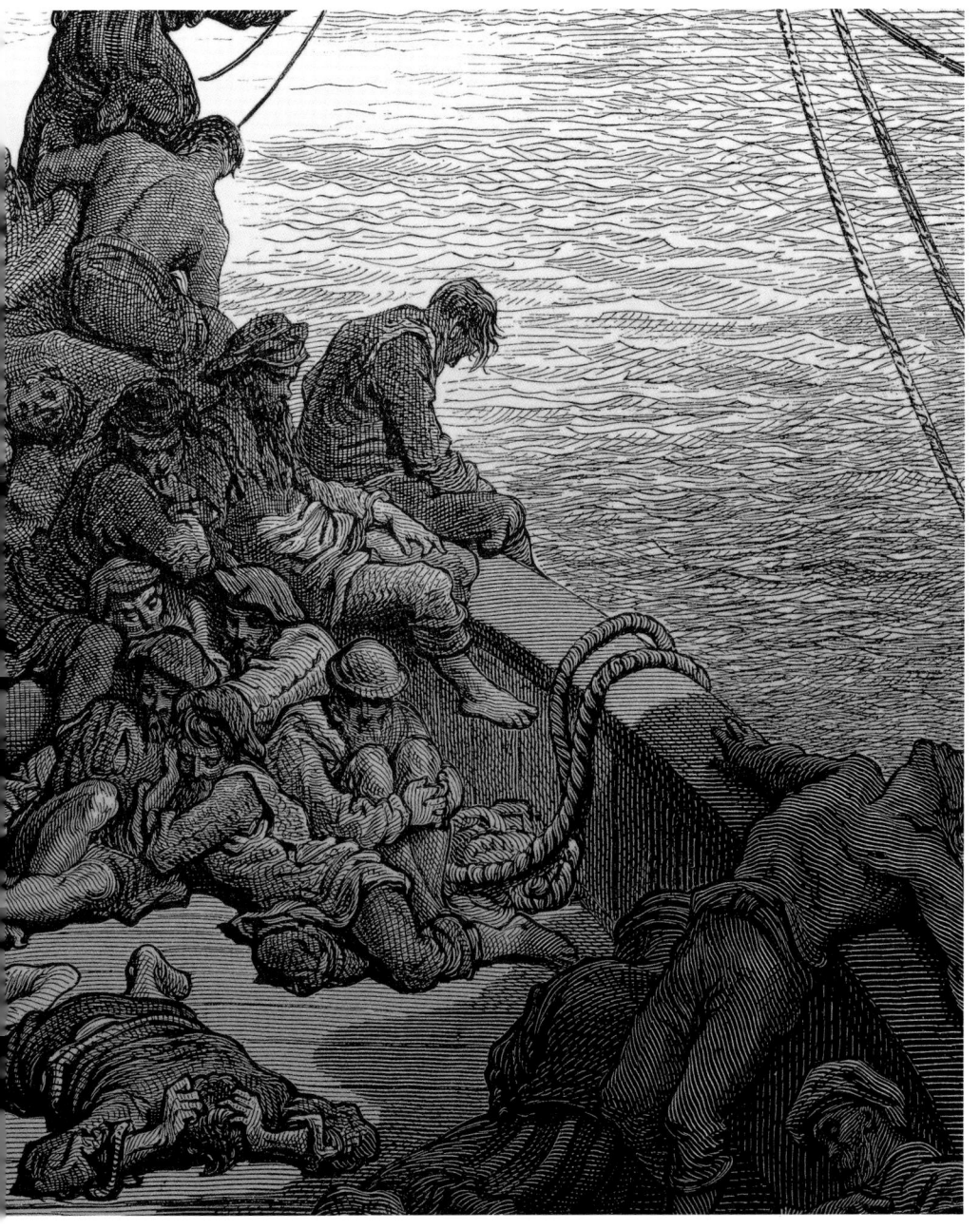

uncommon for sailors, afflicted with scurvy, to walk upon deck, and drop down irrecoverably; though to all appearance, when below there seemed no danger.

Remarkably, old wounds, long healed, were reported to reopen, and once-broken bones were found to re-break.

Alongside the physical characteristics, scurvy also manifested in the mood and behaviour of those afflicted. Trotter and others noted that it was accompanied by exhaustion and melancholy, 'a strange dejection of the spirits [...] and a disposition to be seized with the most dreadful terrors on the slightest accident' (fig. 3). The senses of patients with scurvy (otherwise known as 'scorbutic' patients) were heightened to such an extent that, it was claimed, the sound of a gunshot could be fatal. Smells became overpowering, sights blinding and sounds unbearable. So extreme were these responses that sailors were reported to have literally died from joy at drinking fresh water or eating fruit. Trotter coined the term 'scorbutic nostalgia' to describe the almost unendurable homesickness that attended the disease, with victims experiencing vivid dreams of eating and drinking and home that led to utter despair when they were revealed to be false. Robert Falcon Scott (1868–1912) contracted scurvy during his famous *Discovery* expedition to the Antarctic (1901 –04) and went on to describe the psychological symptoms. In particular, he recounted a longing for seal meat in all its forms; soup made from seal blood, seal liver in porridge, seal blubber. A parliamentary inquiry to investigate an outbreak of scurvy during the British Arctic Expedition of 1875–76 had already suggested that such dreams revealed the body's craving for what it needed most. In this case, though of course it was not understood at the time, Scott dreamed of foods containing vitamin C.

Unlike many diseases, it was possible for a patient with scurvy, even in the later stages, to make a full recovery in a relatively short space of time once they had access to fresh fruits and vegetables. On the other hand, millions of seafarers were not so lucky, and often perished from heart attacks, sometimes merely with the effort it took to climb out of their hammocks. When the corpses of scurvy victims were opened by inquiring surgeons, their bones were found to be black.

We know now that scurvy is caused by a severe deficiency of vitamin C, also known as 'ascorbic acid', though the discovery and isolation of this vital substance was not made until the early 1900s. Unlike most animals, human beings, along with some other species, including guinea pigs and some primates, are unable to make their own vitamin C. As such, they must rely on their diet to provide it. Some foods,

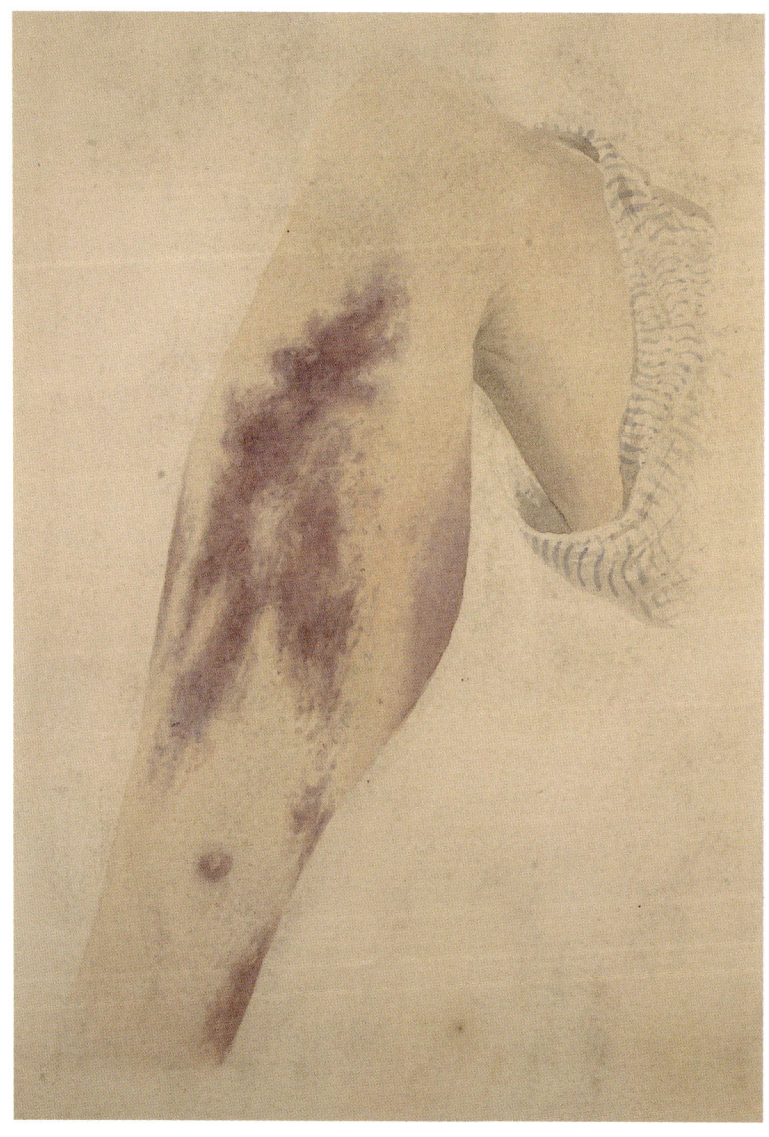

including citrus fruits, broccoli, peppers and other fresh fruits and vegetables are rich in vitamin C. Uncooked, or very lightly cooked, meat is also a good source.

If a person is unable to access these foods, such as while on a ship at sea, then within roughly three to four months the first symptoms of scurvy are likely to appear. We now know that vitamin C is necessary for several vital functions in the body, from the basic structure of our cells to the working of our brains. For instance, vitamin C is essential for the formation of collagen, an important protein which is the primary component of skin, muscles, bones and connective tissue such as ligaments. It is also found in the lining of the intestines and in blood vessels. Without it, cartilage disappears from the joints, bones become fragile, scars reopen and blood vessels weaken and haemorrhage (fig. 4). This explains some of the most obvious symptoms of scurvy, the re-breaking of healed bones, the re-opening of old wounds and the disintegration of the gums and loss of teeth. It also explains why victims might cough up blood, sometimes leading to a misdiagnosis of consumption, or tuberculosis.

Weakened blood vessels trigger haemorrhages, both tiny ones that cause blood blisters to appear around hair follicles, and much larger internal bleeds, which often bring the disease to its conclusion. The haemorrhaging is exacerbated in that

FIG. 4 *Leg from a patient suffering from scurvy*, William Alfred Delamotte, about 1841–51, watercolour, Barts Health NHS Trust Archives

vitamin C also plays a role in the dilation of blood vessels, which allows blood to pass through them easily. Without it, the expansion of the vessels is restricted, causing leakage (fig. 5). In the brain, vitamin C is involved in clearing up waste products and plays a role in the synthesis of important chemicals. When these processes are interrupted, the mood of the patient is affected, as is their sensory perception.

Once you understand the role of vitamin C in the body, it is not hard to recognise how a lack of it causes the profound physical and psychological symptoms of scurvy. The problem is that, for most of human history, nobody had ever heard of vitamin C and so the causes of the disease remained a mystery. From as early as the 1500s, seafarers were reporting that citrus fruits and other fresh foods provided a potent cure for scurvy. Only, no one, from the seafarers themselves to the upper echelons of the medical establishment, knew *why* this was the case, making it almost impossible to forge a unified and appropriate response.

FIG. 5
Leg of a patient with scorbutus (scurvy), unknown artist, 1887, watercolour, Barts Health NHS Trust Archives

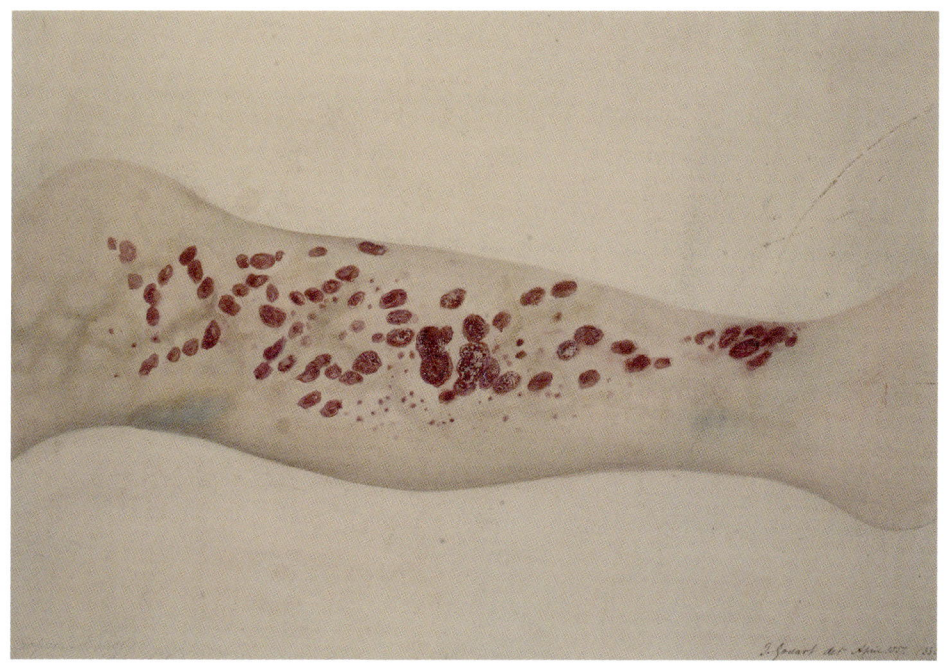

WHAT IS SCURVY?

Chapter 2
A Disease of the Sea

Between 1500 and 1800, scurvy became synonymous with seafaring. The reasons for this are understandable considering the vast changes that took place in the European maritime world during this time, all of which combined to keep ships, and the men on board them, at sea for ever longer durations. Technological developments in shipbuilding and navigation were matched by increased competition to secure trade and colonial territories across the globe. While the Spanish and Portuguese initially dominated southern trading routes to Asia, the French and the British swiftly followed suit and the centre of action for European ships moved from the relatively confined Mediterranean to the vastness of the Atlantic and beyond. In 1497, Portuguese seafarers rounded Cape Horn (the tip of South America), Francis Drake (about 1540–96) led a circumnavigation of the world from 1577–80 and large trading companies, like the East India Company, began widespread voyages to compete with Portuguese and Spanish colonial and trading networks.

The extent of these voyages required longer time away from land, and so the food carried was limited to what could be preserved and stored for significant periods of time. This diet, which was almost entirely devoid of vitamin C, made scurvy inevitable.

Already in 1498, the Portuguese navigator Vasco da Gama (about 1460–1524) reported symptoms identical to scurvy breaking out among his crew around the Cape of Good Hope (the southern tip of Africa). He described the swelling of men's hands and feet and the way their gums grew over their teeth, preventing them from eating. According to his account, their symptoms were eventually alleviated by eating oranges. The Portuguese navigator Ferdinand Magellan (about 1480–1521) reported a similar outbreak during the 1519–22 circumnavigation of the globe, conducted on behalf of Spain. Richard Hawkins (about 1560–1622), writing of his 1593 voyage to the Pacific, described how symptoms of scurvy began around two months after leaving Plymouth in mid-June and how, unable to reach land until mid-October, only four men were still healthy by the time they arrived in Brazil.

At the same time, between the 1500s and 1700s, scurvy was an increasing feature of contemporary medical publications such as *The Surgeon's Mate* (1617) by the first surgeon-general of the East India Company, John Woodall (1570–1643) and

Observationes Circa Scorbutum (1734) by the Dutch surgeon Johann Bachstrom (1688–1742).

A particularly well-known outbreak struck a French expedition led by Jacques Cartier (1491–1557), which sailed for North America in 1535. Three ships left St Malo in May of that year, sailing up the St Lawrence River as far as present-day Quebec and Montreal (fig. 6). The expedition was ultimately forced to spend the winter in the region, and it was in the months that followed that Cartier described an outbreak of scurvy.

> [...] the sickness broke out among us accompanied by the most marvellous and extraordinary symptoms; for some lost all their strength, their legs became swollen and inflamed, while sinews contracted and turned black as coal. In other cases the legs were found blotched with purple-coloured blood. Then the disease would mount to the hips, thighs, shoulders, arms and neck. And all had their mouths so tainted, that the gums rotted away down to the roots of the teeth, which nearly all fell out.

By the middle of February, there were barely ten men in good health, eight were dead and more than 50 were thought likely to die very soon. Assistance came from Domagaya (d. 1539–41), a local Iroquoian and the son of

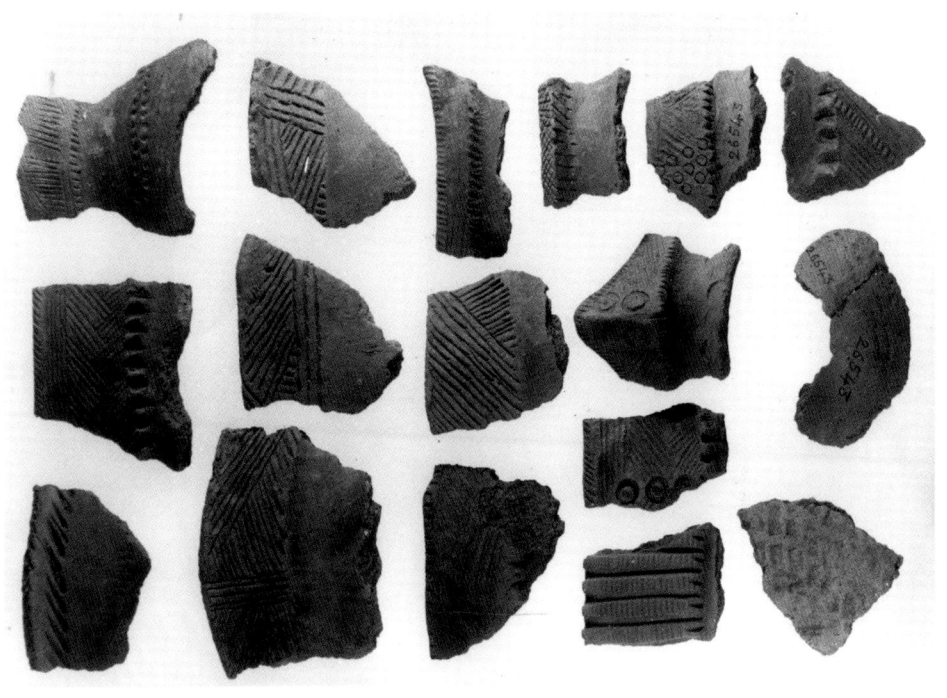

FIG. 6
Pottery shards found on the site of the Iroquoian village, Hochelaga, visited by Jacques Cartier, New York Museum

A DISEASE OF THE SEA

Donnacona (d. 1539–41), chief of the village of Stadacona. The year before, the French and Iroquoian people had come into contact, with relations taking a serious downturn when Cartier erected a large cross in the area. Donnacona was seized and persuaded to allow his sons to travel to France. There is some suggestion in Cartier's writings that scurvy first attacked Stadacona before arriving in the French settlement and that the French forbade the Iroquoians to approach at this time, in case the disease spread to them. Since scurvy is not infectious this proved no defence and, in the end, Domagaya, possibly unwittingly, introduced Cartier and his men to an infusion made from the leaves of a native tree, which was successful in curing the sickness.

For the most part, these early accounts of scurvy relate to commercial and private ventures, but scurvy soon became an important topic in the Royal Navy, as it moved away from coastal defence towards long distance voyages. By the early 1600s, the European maritime nations were engaged in conflicts for control of the seas and oceans, requiring fleets stationed across the world and lengthy blockades of rival ports. In many ways the situation, as relates to scurvy, was worse for these naval ships than for merchant vessels, because without established trading routes, which often included regular stops for restocking supplies, there was no knowing how long it would be between landfalls, or when fresh food could be obtained.

The traditional naval diet was primarily based on salted meat, dried 'pease' (an old spelling of peas) or beans and ships' 'biscuit' (fig. 7). Biscuit, being effectively a hard bread made of flour, water and salt, was a staple of the naval diet though sailors reported that it was regularly infested with weevils, which were removed by tapping or heating before consumption. In 1677, a daily ration for sailors was set at one pound of biscuit and one gallon of beer, and a weekly ration of eight pounds of beef, or four pounds of beef with two of pork or bacon and two pints of pease (fig. 8). In 1733, the Admiralty published its first formal set of regulations for diet at sea, which outlined weekly provisions for each seafarer. They amounted to:

- 7lb (3.2kg) of biscuit
- 7 gallons (32L) of beer
- 4lb (1.8kg) of beef
- 2lb (0.9kg) of pork
- 2lb (0.9kg) of pease
- 3 pints (1.7L) of oatmeal
- 6oz (170g) of butter
- 12oz (340g) of cheese

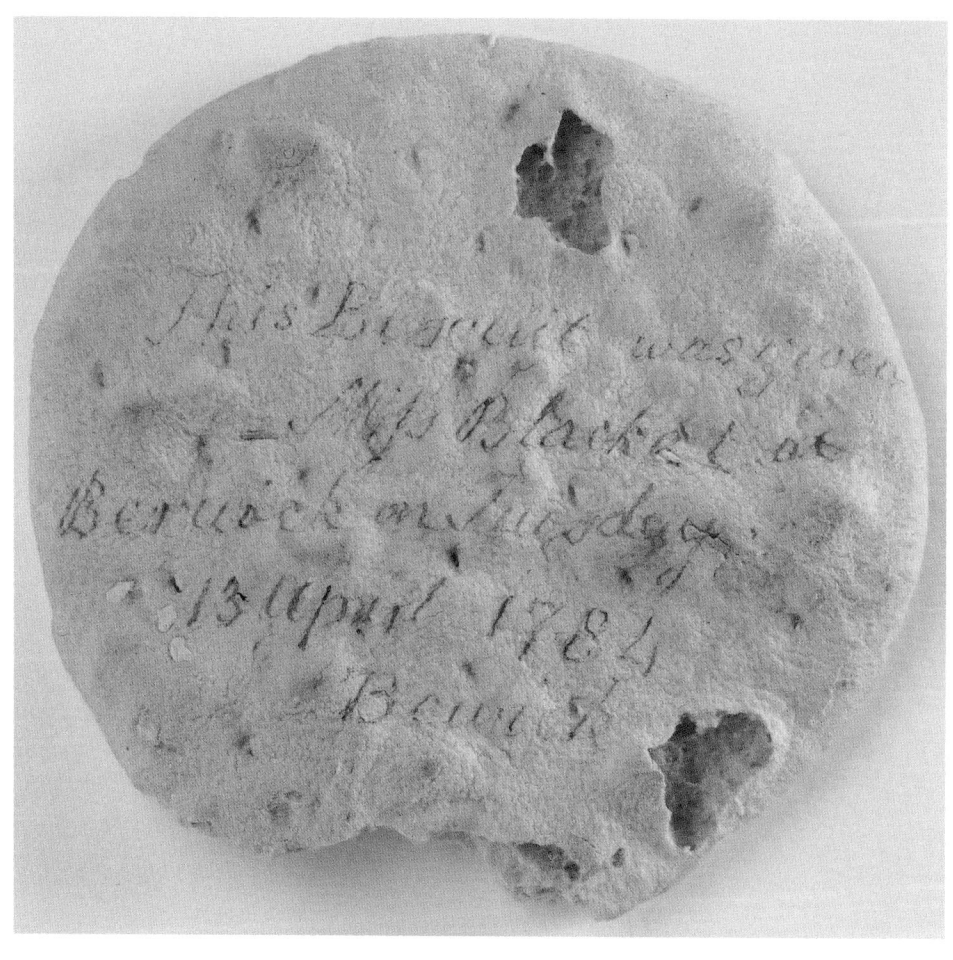

FIG. 7
Ship's biscuit engraved by
Thomas Beswick, 1784,
10 × 95mm, AAB0003

FIG. 8
Victualling account,
1558, CAD/B/1

Hull : Anno 1558

Victuellinge theare for cxx men, mande and provided by watr Johnn and Thomas Alred, Gentyllmen the xxj of May: 1558, and the mony payd vnto them by Edward Bashe, by order of warrant of the Board of thadmyrallte, as folowyth:

The Charite of Hull — be — } xlx Men
The Robart of Hull — be — }

A proportione of victuall allowyd for and towardes the victuallinge of the sayd Shyppes, as folowyth:

Bysquet	...	...
Bere	...	...
Byff	...	...
Stockfishe	...	...
...	...	...
Butter	...	...
Chese	...	...
Cask for Bisquet	...	...
Cask for Biff and water	...	...
Barrells for Butter	...	...
Buckitts for water	...	...
Beare hoyns at the Byginning of the Shyppes	...	...
For lychterage and cariage of the Beare and Biff to Shypbord	...	...
Necessarys to the Pursars after	...	...
For the hyre of ij Sesternes to salte the Biff and making clene of the hoys	...	...
For the Bord wages of xx men xx dayes before theyr entrd into vytellyng	...	...
For the Bord wages of xx men iiij dayes in the maner	...	...

Summa pag

W. Wynter

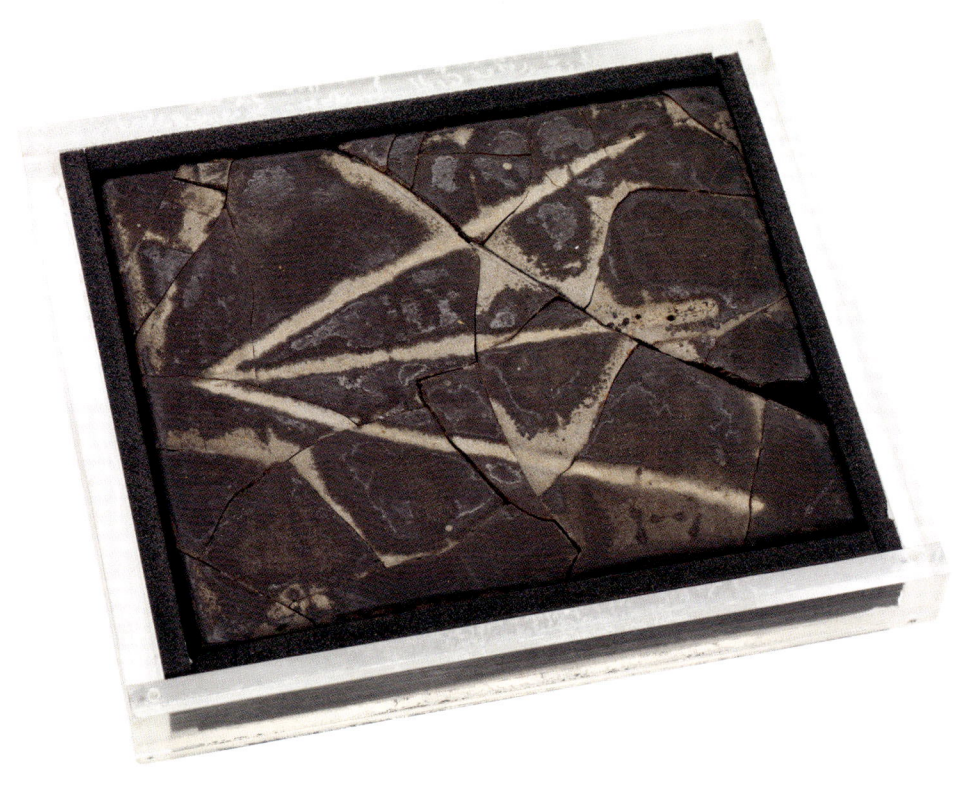

FIG. 9
Portable soup,
mid-to-late 1700s,
5 × 112 × 92mm,
AAB0012

These were to remain little altered until 1847 when canning was adopted. What all of these foodstuffs had in common was a lack of vitamin C.

As scurvy became an increasingly serious problem, especially in the 1700s, efforts were made to improve the seafaring diet. This was not because of any realisation that something vital was missing from it, but rather stemmed from a theory that food that was difficult to digest was the underlying problem. Unfortunately, supplements such as oatmeal, cocoa, rice and sugar, were also devoid of vitamin C and would have no effect. The same was true of another addition, 'portable soup' made from the bones and scraps of meat left from cattle slaughtered for the Navy, which were boiled down and dried. It could then be dissolved in water and consumed (fig. 9). Modern analyses suggest that it would have little to offer as an antiscorbutic, i.e. a treatment for scurvy.

Perhaps the most infamous scurvy-ridden voyage, at least in Britain, was George Anson's (1697–1762) circumnavigation of 1740–44 (figs 10 and 11). Following a declaration of war between Britain and Spain over trade and sovereignty rights in the Caribbean, Anson was ordered by the government to capture the Spanish treasure galleon that sailed annually from Acapulco carrying silver and vast quantities of valuable goods. At the same time, he was to do as much as possible to harass

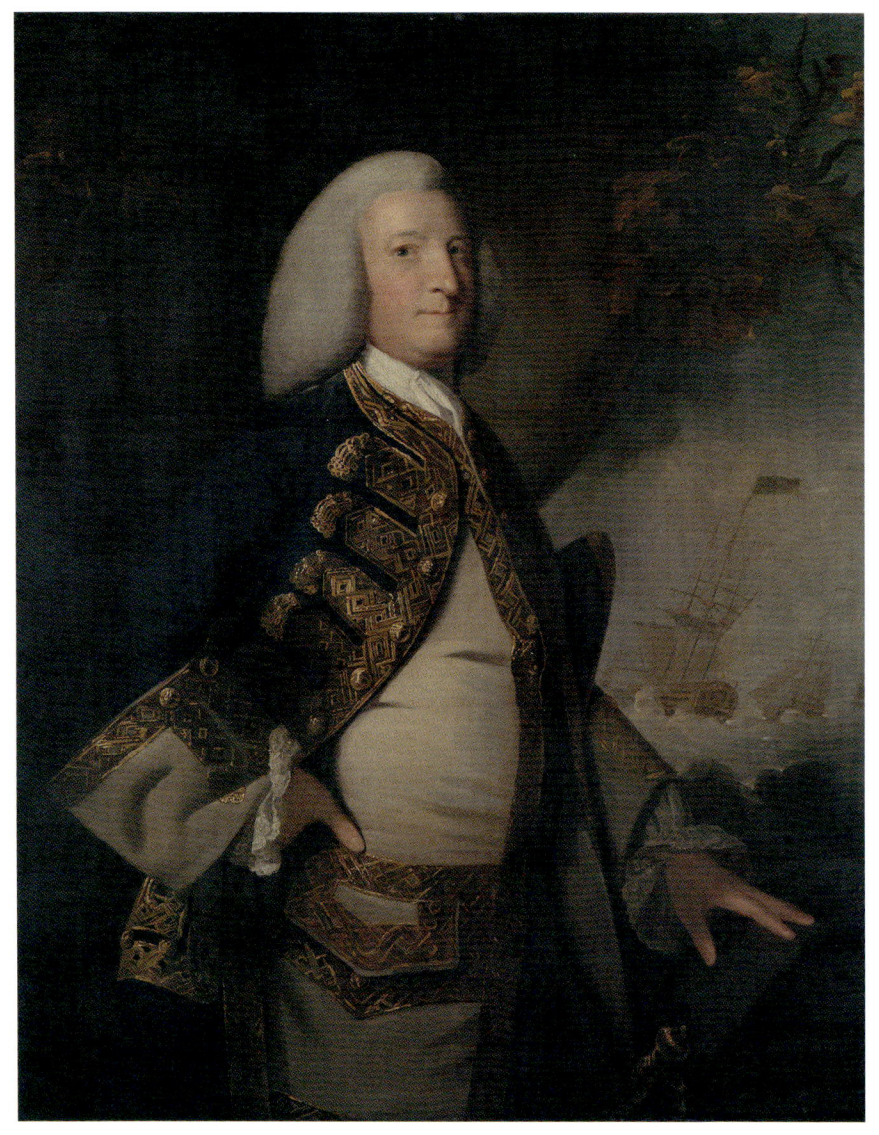

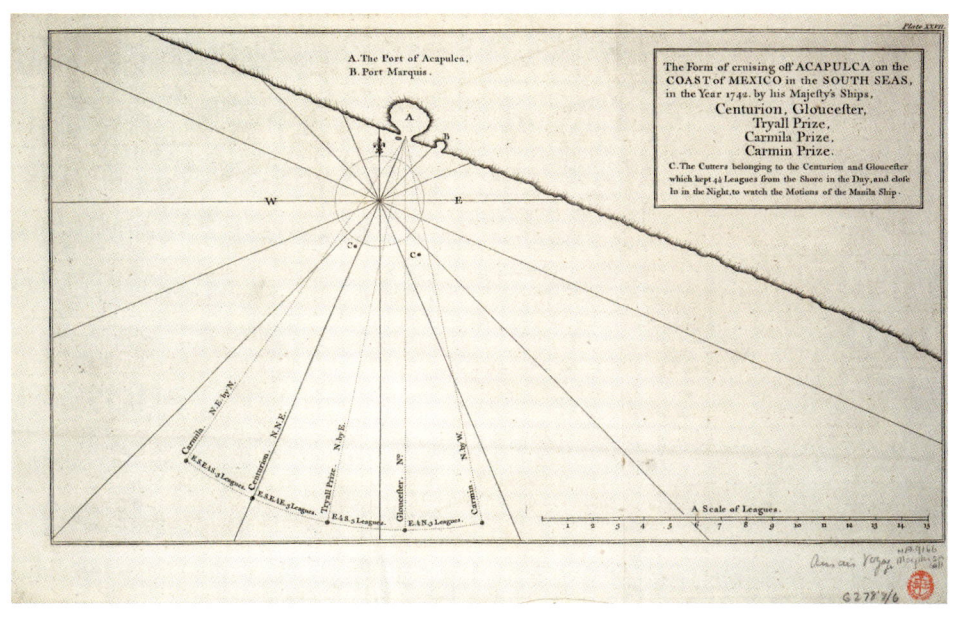

FIG. 10
(OPPOSITE) *Admiral Sir George Anson, 1st Baron Anson (1697–1762)*, in the style of Joshua Reynolds, 1796, oil on canvas, 1,282 × 1,018mm, BHC2516

FIG. 11
The form of cruising off Acapulca on the coast of Mexico in the South Seas, in the year 1742, by His Majesty's ships, 'Centurion', 'Gloucester', 'Tryall Prize', 'Carmila Prize', 'Carmin Prize', George Anson, 1748, chart, 290 × 470mm, G278:8/6

and frustrate Spanish shipping off the west coast of south and central America. The expedition set sail from Spithead in September 1740 and included six warships:

- the flagship *Centurion* (1,005 tons, 60 guns, 400 men)
- *Gloucester* (853 tons, 50 guns, 300 men)
- *Severn* (853 tons, 50 guns, 300 men)
- *Pearl* (600 tons, 40 guns, 250 men)
- *Wager* (599 tons, 24 guns, 120 men)
- *Tryal* (200 tons, eight guns, 70 men)

Two merchant ships, *Anna* and *Industry* would carry provisions.

Four years later, only one ship, *Centurion*, returned and of more than 1,900 men who sailed, around 1,400 had perished. While some of these died of dysentery and even starvation, many lost their lives to scurvy.

The problems began before the expedition even set sail. Many of those on board were in poor health from the start; a severe winter in 1739–40 meant widespread malnutrition among the general population. As was always the case at the start of major wars, there were challenges in manning the fleet, which meant the health of potential crew members was of little consequence. What is more, the long delays in setting sail made the situation worse as men lingered for months waiting for repairs and alterations to the vessels and the requisite number of seamen, all the while living on shipboard rations. Many entered the sick lists before the expedition could even depart.

The situation was so bad that Anson's request for more men was met in August 1740 with pensioners from Chelsea Hospital. Instead of the regiment of regular soldiers which he had been expecting, the pensioners were former servicemen who had been determined unfit for duty by virtue of age, illness or wounds and, the surviving records suggest, their average age was around 55. Among their complement was Charles Ross, aged 53, suffering with fits and difficulty with hearing, and Edward Butler, aged 70, who had a 'hurt' in his back and was 'worn out'. They had little chance of survival and by October 1742 only one of the 40 who sailed on the flagship was still alive. All 60 who embarked on *Gloucester* were dead by mid-1741. In the muster book for the *Centurion,* there is a list of some of the 'invalids' who boarded in August 1740 along with their fates. 'Charles Ross' appears towards the bottom of the page. He is listed as 'DD' or 'discharged dead' on 20 June 1741, his body apparently left in the San Fernandez Islands in the Pacific (fig. 12). A contingent of marines was also sent to boost numbers, but these were mostly raw recruits, often young and sickly, who had never so much as fired a gun. The

Number	Entry	Date	Whence	Ticket	Name & Quality	on R	Docket	Qual.	Whither	Topsellers the supplied 2/9 of the Dockers Order	Ditto
356		5 Augt 1740	Invalids		Nichd Terrill	D	18 April 1740		Sea		0.9.6
					Geo. Shaft	D	0 Augt 1740	1			
					Richd Hetherington	D	9 May 1741		Sea		0.9.6
					Thos Hatfield	D	0 Augt 1740				
360					Jno Hughes	D	4 May 1741		Sea		0.9.6
					Wm Hill	D	0 Augt 1740		Sea		0.9.6
					Andw Johnson	D	29 May 1741		Sea		0.9.6
					Patk Jones						
					Josh Jones	}	8 August 1740				
5					Jno Kelley						
					Joseph Lewis						
					Alexr McDonald	D	10 April 1741		Sea		0.9.6
					Daniel McMichael	D	22 Do	Do			0.9.6
					Neel McNeal	D	3 Feb 1740	Do			0.9.6
370					Thos Mills	D	0 Do Do	Do			0.9.6
					Jno Murray	D	19 April 1741	Do			0.9.6
					Daniel Marcey	D	9 Jant 1740		Whither		0.9.6
					Wm York	D	11 Augt 1740				
					Richd Parsthouse	D	18 Do 1740		Sea		0.9.6
5					Wm Peachey	D	8 August 1740				
					Samt Pryer	D	7 Feby 1740		Sea		0.9.6
					Christr Pitty	D	8 Augt 1740				
					Charles Ross	D	20 June 1741		Fernando		0.9.6
					James Samuell	D	11 Feb 1740		Sea		0.9.6
380					Robt Savory	D	11 April 1741		Sea		0.9.6
					Jno Smith	D	0 Augt 1740				
					Hugh Smith	D	1 May 1741		Sea		0.9.6
					Thos Steers	D	5 Do Do	Do			0.9.6
					Wm Thompson	D	0 Augt 1740	Do			

marines, like the pensioners, quickly fell ill. By mid-1741 only 13 of the 82 who sailed on *Centurion* were alive.

Scurvy was a well-known factor in long voyages at this time and so Anson's ships were supplied with preventatives and treatments. Unfortunately, these provisions were totally ineffective. The 'elixir of vitriol' recommended by the Royal College of Physicians was comprised of sulphuric acid mixed with alcohol, sugar and spices. On top of this, the Navy Board issued a well-known medicine, Ward's drop and pill. Invented by Joshua Ward (1684/5–1761), the 'pill' contained antimony (a chemical element) and some form of vegetable and wine, while the 'drop' was comprised of nitric acid, ammonium chloride and mercury. Both remedies resulted in sweating and significant gastrointestinal symptoms, likely to have weakened anyone already ill further. The ships were also provided with tamarinds, a fruit in the pea family, seemingly at Anson's request. While tamarinds do contain vitamin C, it is unlikely they could have been preserved for any meaningful duration and therefore would have been of limited value as a preventative for scurvy.

The ships finally left Britain in September 1740, and by spring the following year, found themselves battling both ferocious storms around Cape Horn and the first outbreaks of scurvy. The best-selling authorised account of the expedition,

FIG. 12 Detail of *Centurion* muster roll, 1 July 1739–30 September 1741, The National Archives, London

A Voyage Around the World by George Anson (1748) states:

> [...] the scurvy began to make its appearance amongst us; and our long continuance at sea, the fatigue we underwent, and the various disappointments we met with, had occasioned its spreading to such a degree, that at the latter end of April there were but few on board, who were not in some degree afflicted with it, and in that month no less than forty three died of it on board the *Centurion*.

The problem soon worsened, 'double that number' were lost in May and the situation remained dreadful in June, so that by the middle of that month they had lost more than 200 men. The pensioners suffered particularly badly as old wounds reopened. One man found that his leg, which had been broken at the Battle of the Boyne (1690), fractured again and previously healed wounds from the same battle re-emerged.

Of the six warships, only *Centurion*, *Gloucester* and *Tryal*, along with the merchant ship *Anna*, made it to the San Fernandez Islands in the Pacific, where their crews were able to recover their strength with access to fresh fruits, vegetables and fish. Nonetheless, by the time they left, two thirds of those who had set sail in the three warships in 1740 were dead, with only 335 of 961 men still alive. There were enough men to sail the remaining ships, but not enough to fight and while prisoners from Spanish ships briefly bolstered numbers, these men were later released. Another 43 prisoners, including enslaved peoples, were kept on board. By the time the expedition headed westward into the Pacific, there were only enough men for *Centurion* and *Gloucester* to continue. *Tyral* had been scuttled after damage inflicted during the pursuit of the Spanish merchant ship *Arranzazu* but this and other Spanish prizes had to be abandoned.

The surgeon on board *Centurion*, Harry Ettick, had blamed the initial outbreak of scurvy on the cold climate, which he believed affected the blood, making it too thin for proper circulation. But he was left without answers when scurvy once again broke out during the incredibly slow journey across the Pacific. As Pascoe Thomas, the schoolmaster on *Centurion* wrote, 'But this passage, in a very hot climate, where the symptoms were not only more dreadful, but the mortality much more quick and fatal in proportion to the number of people, put our scheming doctor to a sad nonplus; he could not account for this.'

Ettick came instead to the conclusion that scurvy was simply caused by too long at sea, and that, as Thomas recorded, 'no other cure but the shore should ever take place.'

Thomas himself was struck down in July 1742:

> I was first taken about the beginning of the month with a small pain on the joint of my left great toe […] in a little time a large black spot appearing on the part affected, with very intense pains at the bone […] several hard nodes began to rise in my legs, thighs and arms, and not only many more black spots appeared in the skin, but those spread […] and this accompanied with such excessive pains in the joints of the knees, ankles and toes, as I thought, before I experienced them, that human nature could ever have supported. It next advanced to my mouth; all my teeth were presently loose, and my gums, overcharged with extravasated blood, fell down quite almost over my teeth. This occasioned my breath to stink much, yet without affecting my lungs; but I believe, one more week at sea would have ended me.

Many would perish from the disease and by the end of August, when the remaining sailors arrived on Tinian, an island in the Marianas chain, *Gloucester* had also been abandoned. The ship was badly damaged and by the middle of the month, out of 97 on board, only 16 men and 11 boys were in a fit state to sail. By the time they reached land, even the healthiest were so weak that after carrying the sick ashore, they were unable to tend to them. Thomas wrote that after being dropped on the ground, many were physically unable to reach supplies of fruit or water even where they were only yards away. Thankfully, the island provided bountiful fruits and vegetables that allowed many to regain their health.

Centurion set sail again in October and at last arrived in Macao, a Portuguese settlement at the time, where the ship could undergo desperately needed repairs before setting out once more in pursuit of the Spanish treasure galleon. By this time there were only 227 on board, a number which included several young boys and some Dutch seamen and lascars taken on at Macao. The latter is a broad term for sailors from the Indian Ocean. In June that year, *Centurion* finally took the *Nuestra de Señora de Covadonga* and returned to Britain with an enormous haul of riches (fig. 13).

Despite the so-called 'success' of the expedition, the vast mortality rate proved an extraordinary shock to the nation. There was also a considerable financial cost, as the abandonment of ships like *Gloucester* presented a huge loss on Admiralty investment. But it was partly the news of Anson's expedition that prompted the Scottish surgeon James Lind's (1716–94) attempt to find an effective cure for this vicious disease, responsible for such significant loss of life at sea.

FIG. 13 *The Capture of the 'Nuestra Señora de Cavadonga' by the 'Centurion', 20 June 1743*, Samuel Scott, about 1745, oil on canvas, 1,029 × 1,511mm, BHC0360

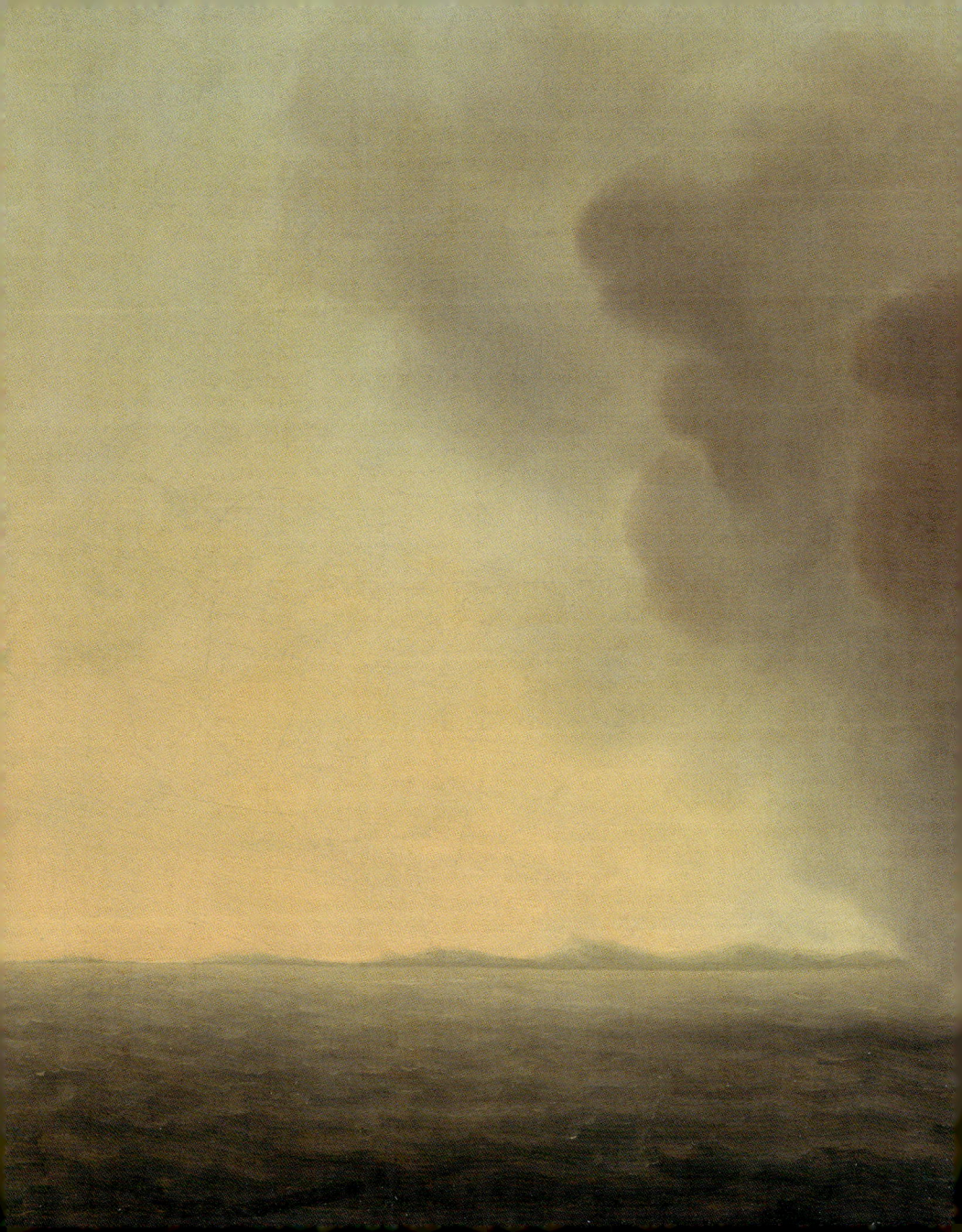

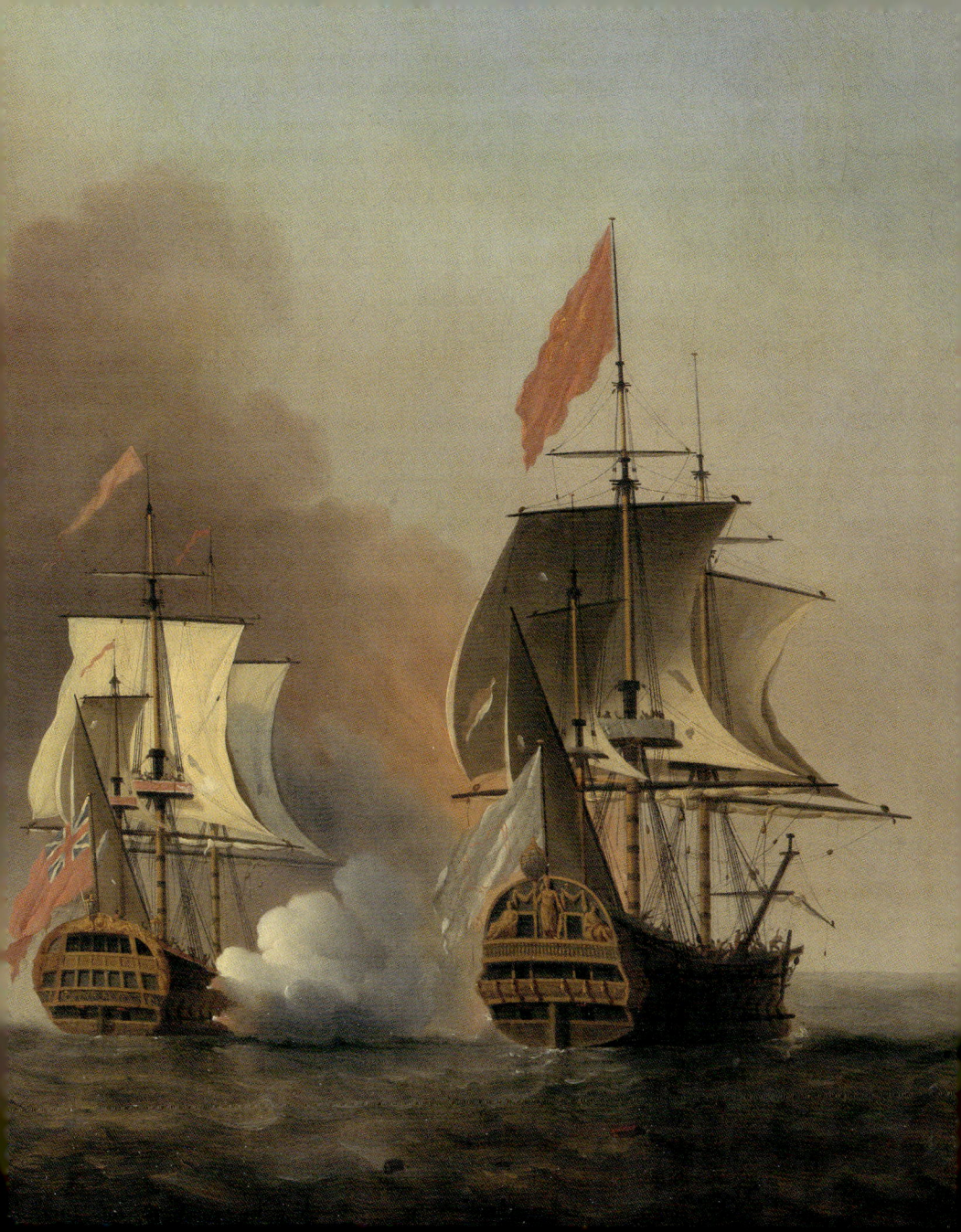

Chapter 3
The Search for a Cure

As early as 1498, evidence had suggested that fresh fruits and vegetables, and especially citrus, acted as a potent cure for scurvy. The journals of James Lancaster (1554/5–1618) and Richard Hawkins (about 1560–1622), written in the sixteenth and seventeenth centuries, had already recommended their use, corroborating accounts of seafarers such as Vasco da Gama in the late fifteenth century. In 1607 the East India Company included 'lemon water' in the supplies for future expeditions, though the quantities do not seem to have been recorded. Similarly, the Dutch East India Company sought to establish orchards and vegetable gardens along their trade routes, and some ships even tried to grow gardens on deck, though this proved impractical. In *The Surgeons Mate* (1617), John Woodall (1570–1643) recommended a good quantity of lemon juice to be sent on each ship for the relief of scorbutic sailors and even made reference to surgeons who administered the juice daily, by way of prevention.

The question then is why this did not lead to the universal adoption and provision of such foodstuffs to prevent the disease breaking out at sea. The answers are varied and complicated but perhaps not incomprehensible in a world with no knowledge of vitamin C's existence, let alone its impact on the body and mind. The problem lay in large part in the difficulty of provisioning large ships for such long durations, since fresh foods do not keep over significant periods. Added to this, later attempts to concentrate and preserve the juice of citrus fruits substantially reduced their levels of vitamin C, making them less effective and calling their value into question.

The difference in status between ships' surgeons and land-based physicians meant the latter were ultimately relied upon for solutions to the problem, despite their lack of seagoing experience. This meant that advice tended to be based on the medical fashions or theories of the day, or the most powerful voices, rather than on empirical evidence. Much medical practice in the period when scurvy was at its most widespread relied on the ideas of ancient thinkers such as Galen (about 129–about 216/17) and Hippocrates (about 460 BCE–about 370 BCE). It was suggested that health rested on a balance, and poor health on an imbalance, of four bodily humours: blood, phlegm, black bile and yellow bile. So wedded were they to these ancient ideas that physicians such as John

Echth (about 1515–54), writing in 1541, were able to argue that those with an excess of black bile may contract scurvy without any external factors present at all. Scurvy was also associated strongly with damage to the spleen, possibly resulting from dietary factors, particularly the salt meat and stale water consumed at sea.

Another idea advocated by medical professionals suggested that there were two forms of the disease: one caused by food turning acidic in the stomach, and another resulting from food that turned alkaline. There were even theories that scurvy was a venereal disease or that sailors who were idle were most likely to succumb. The latter was particularly problematic since the onset of the disease was often accompanied by fatigue and exhaustion, so that sailors who were already unwell were pushed ever harder in a counterintuitive effort to keep them healthy. Confusion as to the cause of scurvy led to an array of possible treatments. While John Woodall argued for citrus as a cure for scurvy, he also advocated oil of vitriol as an effective alternative. Some physicians even recommended hydrochloric acid and others went so far as to suggest citrus fruit should be avoided since it was liable to result in fevers and damage to vital organs.

Scottish surgeon James Lind took a more experimental approach in his search for a cure (fig. 14). Born in Edinburgh

FIG. 14 *Portrait of James Lind (1716–94)*, G. Chalmers and I. Wright, 1932, engraving, 120 × 165mm, Wellcome Collection

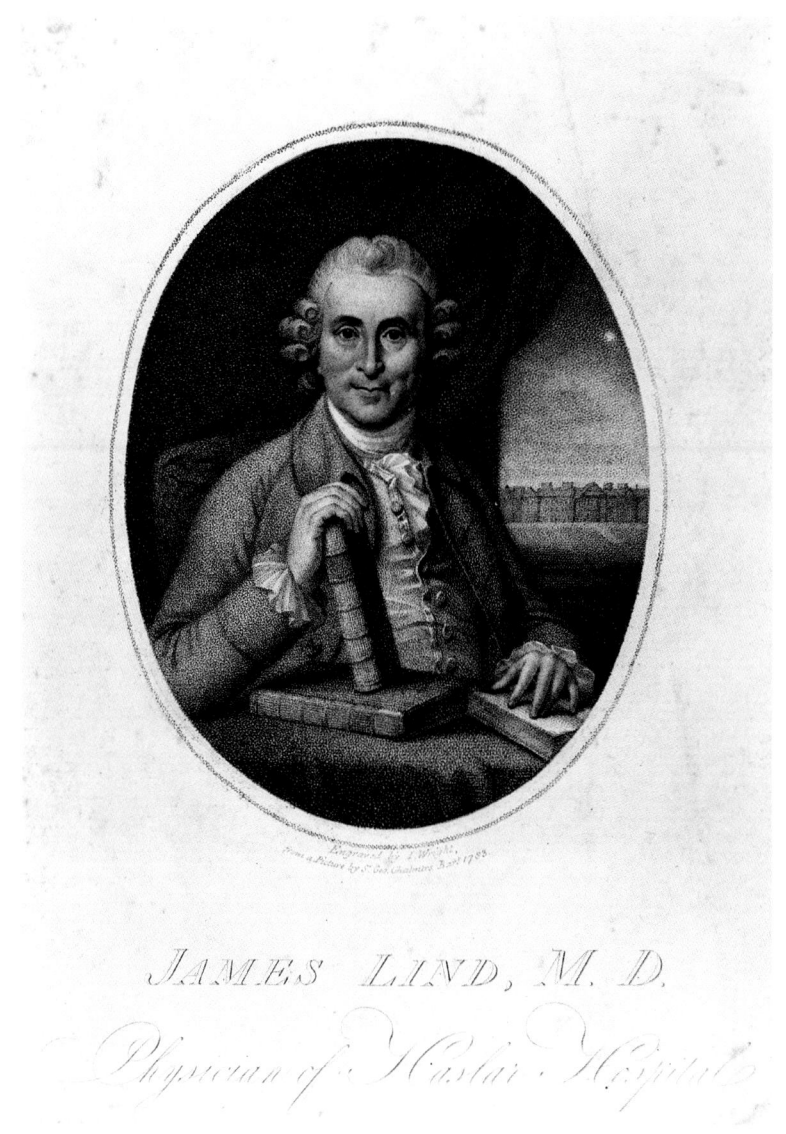

JAMES LIND, M.D.
Physician of Haslar Hospital

to a merchant family, Lind went on to work as a surgeon in the Royal Navy, serving on board HMS *Salisbury* in the Channel during the summer of 1747. It was there that he witnessed a serious outbreak of scurvy, precipitating what is considered to be 'the first controlled trial in clinical nutrition' ever mounted. Lind took 12 sailors suffering from scurvy and divided them into six groups. They were kept in the same quarters and given the same diet: fresh mutton broth, puddings, barley, raisins, currants, rice and so on. Then each of the groups was given a different daily treatment over the course of 14 days. These different treatments were as follows:

- Group 1: a quart (1.1 litres) of cider.
- Group 2: 25 drops of elixir of vitriol, three times a day.
- Group 3: 6 spoonfuls of vinegar, three times a day.
- Group 4: half a pint (approximately 0.3 litres) of seawater
- Group 5: two oranges and one lemon a day, though this was curtailed after six days when supplies ran out.
- Group 6: a paste made of garlic, mustard seed, balsam of Peru (tree resin), horseradish, and gum myrrh. In addition, barley water, made more acidic by the addition of tamarinds, and on some occasions with cream of tartar.

Knowing what we know now, the results should be easy to predict. Those who received lemons and oranges recovered to such an extent after six days that they were well enough to assist in nursing the other patients. Group 1, who received cider, showed some recovery after two weeks but the others showed no improvement at all. Lind could conclude that oranges and lemons were the most effective cures for scurvy at sea.

Lind left the Navy the following year, whereupon he became a licensed physician and, in 1750, was elected as a Fellow of Edinburgh's Royal College of Physicians. In 1753 he published *A Treatise on the Scurvy* in which he outlined his thoughts on the disease and insisted on the importance of evidence in support of theory (fig. 15). Yet, remarkably, the results of his trial seem to have had little impact on the fight against the disease and his own conclusions remained somewhat unfocused. Lind did not believe, despite the result of his experiment, that there was anything specific in fresh fruit that prevented scurvy, rather that it worked as a treatment for a disease arising from other causes. Likewise, he did not believe it to be the only cure, but rather one of a number of which it was simply the most effective.

His own theory was based on a popular idea of the eighteenth century: the concept of 'blocked perspiration'. Physicians supposed, drawing on ancient medical theories, that perspiration, or sweating, was a major route for the

A TREATISE ON THE SCURVY.

IN THREE PARTS.

CONTAINING

An Inquiry into the Nature, Causes, and Cure, of that Disease.

Together with

A Critical and Chronological View of what has been published on the Subject.

By *JAMES LIND*, M.D.

Fellow of the Royal College of Physicians in *Edinburgh*.

The SECOND EDITION corrected, with Additions and Improvements.

LONDON:
Printed for A. MILLAR in the *Strand*.
MDCCLVII.

removal of unwanted vapours and humours from the body. Without this escape, the vapours built up and became putrid and corrupted, resulting in a variety of diseases. Lind believed that the cold, damp environment at sea blocked perspiration and so contributed to outbreaks of scurvy. As such, he suggested, lemons and limes worked as a cure because they were able to break down digestive products that resulted from a shipboard diet, which would otherwise become harmful. For Lind, diet *and* moisture were causes of the disease. He even suggested that scurvy could be divided into two types, one occurred because a person was exposed to the wrong conditions while the other resulted from an inherent disposition towards the illness. While he recognised, to some extent, that diet was a factor in outbreaks of scurvy, he did not believe that it was the automatic outcome of long incidence without access to fresh fruits and vegetables. He was able to point to northern countries where people were deprived of such foods for much of the winter without scurvy being commonplace. He was clearly failing to take into account root vegetables such as potatoes, which we now know do contain vitamin C. Despite the results of his experiment, Lind fell into a common trap of the time, in ascribing to scurvy numerous causes and potential cures, rather than the simple, singular one that his results implied.

FIG. 15 Title page from *A Treatise on the Scurvy, in three parts. Containing an inquiry into the nature, causes, and cure, of that disease. Together with a critical and chronological view of what has been published on the subject*, James Lind, originally published 1753, A. Miller, London

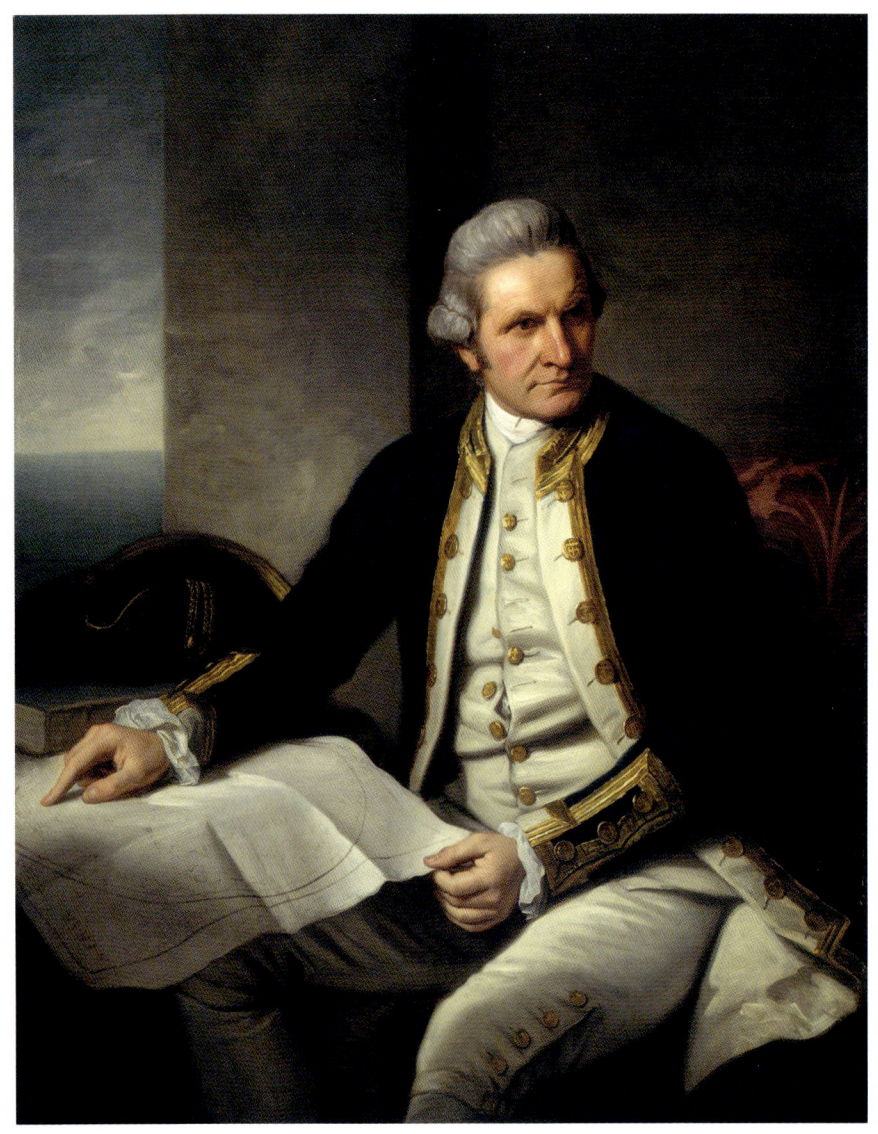

Lind did recommend a technique for preserving the juice of oranges and lemons for sea voyages in a syrup known as 'rob'. Unfortunately, the techniques for making rob, which involved evaporating the juice down to a tiny quantity of its initial volume, also resulted in significant loss of vitamin C. It is now also known that storing the rob for any considerable period of time led to further reduction of ascorbic acid. Since it would not realistically have been given to sailors until they were already suffering from scurvy, likely after months at sea, it is not surprising that the Sick and Hurt Board (the commissioners responsible for the welfare of sick and wounded sailors), considered the rob to be of no use in the treatment of the disease.

Lind attempted further experiments at Haslar Royal Naval Hospital near Portsmouth, where he had been appointed physician in 1758. The results, however, appear to have been somewhat confused and complicated by contradictory evidence. There were even claims that men who had been living on salted meats remained in good health, only succumbing to scurvy after arriving in port and eating ripe fruits and green vegetables. Lind eventually came to conclude, in the final edition of his *Treatise* (1772), that cold air, damp accommodation and confinement combined with the want of green vegetables were the common causes of

FIG. 16 *Captain James Cook (1728–79)*, Nathaniel Dance, 1775–6, oil on canvas, 1,270 × 1,016mm, BHC2628

scurvy. Though he suggested that confinement was the most important factor, he did advise that a syrup of lemons should always be carried by surgeons at sea. He was also honest that his work remained imperfect and his proposals uncertain.

It seems that while there was a growing consensus that eating fresh fruit and vegetables would cure scurvy, this did not automatically equate to the belief that deficient diet caused the disease, or at least not on its own. Further experiments were carried out at sea, including during Captain James Cook's (1728–79, fig. 16) famous voyage to the Pacific in *Endeavour* in the years 1768-71. Cook's orders from the Admiralty included observing the time and transit of Venus in June 1769, charting the coastline of New Zealand and establishing the presence, or not, of a 'Great Southern Continent'. But he was also given instructions to carry a variety of antiscorbutic foodstuffs and to report on their efficacy. These were: sauerkraut, portable soup, saloup (a jelly like substance made from the roots of orchids), malt and rob of oranges and lemons. In an extract from the journal of HMS *Endeavour,* Cook writes:

> In the PM saild the Holton Indiaman who saluted us with 11 Guns, which Compliment we returnd. This Ship during her stay in India lost by sickness between 30 and 40 Men and had at this time a good ma[n]y down with the

scurvy. Other ships suffer'd as much or more by Sickness than we have done who have been out near three times as long (fig. 17).

Over the three-year expedition not one man died of scurvy, nor was anyone seriously ill with it. It should be noted, however, that, unlike in the ordinary fleet, all of the men were hand selected and they were never away from land for longer than around 17 weeks. At each landing, Cook secured provisions of fresh fruit and vegetables and made sure the men ate them. With such a range of measures, it was impossible to tell exactly which had been effective and so while Cook argued at one point that sauerkraut had been of particular importance, the surgeon's mate emphasised the value of malt. Joseph Banks (1743–1820), the naturalist on board *Endeavour* and later president of the Royal Society, recorded that he had in fact felt some early signs of the disease, and it was lemon juice which provided the cure. Nonetheless, a year later, he promoted wort, the liquid produced from ground malt, as of equal virtue to fresh vegetables and one of the most potent treatments against scurvy.

Cook's next expedition (1772–75) was once more in search of the Great Southern Continent. Again, he was supplied with a range of antiscorbutic foods including:

Cape of Good Hope —

Saturday 16: March 1776 Variable light airs all this da[y]
Moor'd the Ship and struck yards and topmast[s]
and in the Morning got all the Sick [28] ashor[e]
to quarters provided for them and got fres[h]
meat and greens for the people on board —

Sunday 17 In the am sail'd for England the
Admiral Pocock, Capt. Riddel, by whom I sen[t]
letters to the Admiralty & Royal Society. About
Noon came on a hard dry gale from the SE

Monday 18 In the PM anchor'd in the offi[ng]
the Holton Indiaman an English Ship which
prov'd to be the Holton Indiaman from Ben[gal]
In the am it fell moderate and we began to d[o?]
the Ship

Tuesday 19 Variable gentle breezes all this da[y]
Employ'd repairing sails, rigging, watering &c

Wednesday 20: In the PM sail'd the Holton Ind[iaman]
who saluted us with a 11 guns, which complimen[t we]
return'd. This Ship during her stay in India los[t]
by sickness between 30 and 40 Men and had a[t]
this time a good many down with the scurvy, othe[r]
Ships suffer'd in the same proportion. thus we fin[d]
that Ships which have been little more than 12 [?]
Months from England have suffer'd as much o[r]
more by sickness than we have done who ha[ve]
been out near three times as long, yet their
sufferings will hardly be mention'd in England

when on the other hand those of the Endeavour being
the Vessels is uncommon, will very probable be
mentioned in every News paper and what is not
unlikely with many additional hardships we
never experienced for such are the dispositions
of men in general in these Voyages that they
are seldom content with the hardships and dangers
which will naturaly occur, but they must add
others which hardly ever had existence but in their
imaginations by magnifying the most trifling
accidents and circumstances to the greatest hardships
and unsurmountable dangers without the imediate
interposition of Providence as if the whole merit
of the Voyage consisted in the dangers and hardships
they underwent, or that real ones did not happen
often enough to give the mind sufficient anxiety,
thus posterity are taught to look upon their Voyages
as hazardous to the highest degree

Thursday 21st Fine pleasant weather, Employ'd
giting on board water, overhauling the riging
and repairing Sails — Sail'd for Batavia a Dutch
Ship —

Friday 22d } Mostly fine pleasant weather, on
Saturday 23d the 23d we compleated our
Sunday 24   water after which I gave as many
Monday 25   of the people leave to go ashore to
Tuesday 26   refresh themselves as could be
             spared at one time —

- sauerkraut
- salted cabbage
- portable soup
- malt (barley or another grain that has been specially prepared for use in brewing and distilling)
- saloup
- mustard
- instructions for making soda water (water with 'fixed air', i.e. carbon dioxide)
- rob of oranges and lemons
- carrot marmalade

Once again, Cook returned without losses to scurvy. In a report to the Royal Society in 1776, he stressed the importance of wort, though he clarified that he did not believe it would be effective where scurvy was already in an advanced state. He also argued for the value of sauerkraut and portable soup, noting that the latter was often served with fresh vegetables. Finally, though he recognised that the rob had been useful in some cases, he emphasised the value of sugar, fresh water and general cleanliness. As with his earlier voyage, it is clear to see the difficulty in forming conclusions from so many methods tested simultaneously. Cook did however

FIG. 17 (PREVIOUS) Extract from the journal of HMS *Endeavour*, Captain James Cook, 1768–1771, JOD/19

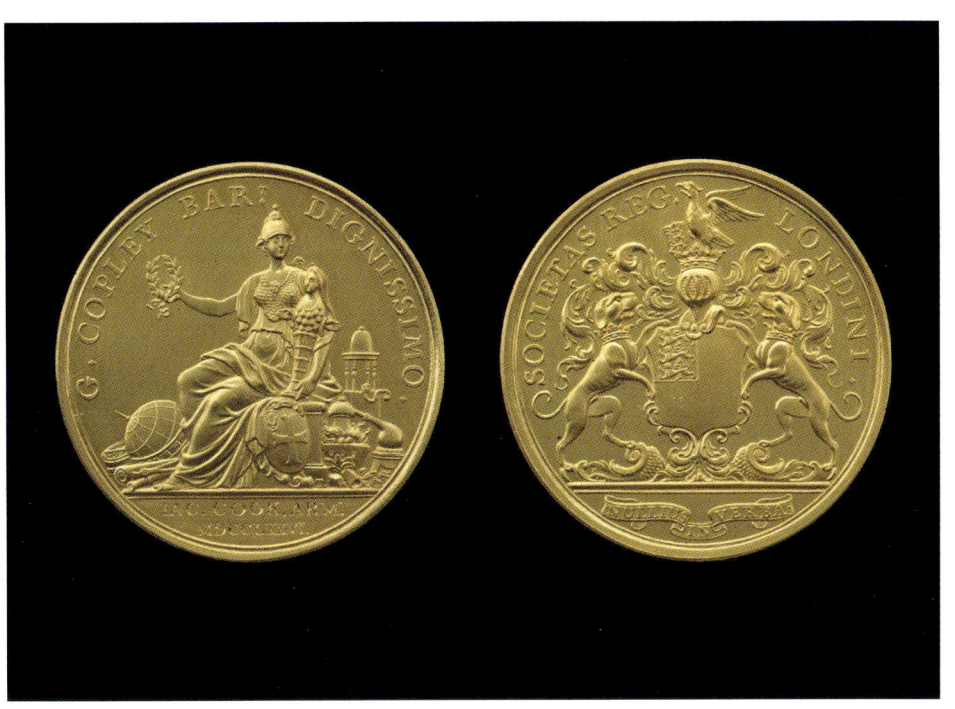

FIG.18 Copley Medal awarded to Captain James Cook, 1776, gold, British Museum

receive the Copley Medal, awarded by the Royal Society for sustained and outstanding achievement in any scientific field, for keeping his voyages scurvy free (fig. 18).

Despite Cook's account, which implied a range of measures were effective against scurvy and cast some doubt on the efficacy of malt, the latter was wholeheartedly embraced as the chief antiscorbutic at sea in the following decades. This even though we now know malt has no value in the prevention and treatment of scurvy. There is reason to believe that the official promotion of malt over lemons and limes had more to do with cost and the politics of the medical establishment than any real therapeutic benefit. Influential figures in the medical establishment who were already persuaded as to the value of malt may have seized on Cook's successes to push forward their favoured remedy. Likewise, concerns over the price of citrus may have made malt attractive, with the added benefit that it could be stored and preserved over a long period.

Various theories were mooted as to why malt should be effective. It was proposed that, as malt was used to make liquid wort, which could in turn be fermented and used to make beer, so wort would ferment in the bodies of scorbutic sailors and counter the internal putrefaction that was believed to cause the disease. Interestingly, proponents of this theory argued that fresh vegetables could have the same effect but were simply not practical on long voyages. It is possible that wort did have an effect on sailors who were suffering from a different deficiency, notably in niacin, or vitamin B3, which can be found in malt. Known as pellagra, the resulting illness causes skin problems, diarrhoea and dementia-like symptoms, as well as a swaying walk and blackened tongue and in some cases may have been mistaken for scurvy. In an earlier essay on the means of preventing scurvy at sea, written around 1770, the author promotes the 'good effects' of hop beer in the prevention and cure of scurvy. That his own concern may not be purely for the seafarers is clear as he suggests that: 'should this scheme contribute to the preservation of the health of our brave seamen, promote the interests of the hop and sugar planters and add to the public reserve, it is humbly hoped the author of it will be thought to merit some share of favour' (fig. 19).

Another important figure in the fight against scurvy was Scottish surgeon Thomas Trotter (fig. 20). Trotter began his career at sea in 1779 as a surgeon's mate, encountering scurvy almost immediately and even suffering from it himself. In 1783, unable to find work in the Royal Navy, he joined *Brooks*, a ship which was to transport enslaved African people across the Atlantic. Scurvy broke out among the captives, those whom Trotter had initially described as 'young, stout, and apparently healthy'. But their diet, consisting of 'beans, rice, and Indian

The good Effects of the Hop Beer as recommended in the following Essay are founded in Reason, and have been confirmed by Experience in the follo— Diseases, Viz. in the Muriatic Scurvy, or that Species of Scurvy with whi— Seamen are peculiarly Afflicted, in the Dropsy, Jaundice, and Œdemato— Swellings, Succeeding Malignant Fevers, and Fevers of long Continuan—

It is apprehended, the greatest difficulty to prove the Utility of H— Beer, and the Alterations in Seamens Diet, mentioned in the Essay, is to o— a fair trial at Sea; It is well known how prevalent Custom is, and how ha— we are brought to break thro' Habits which have the Sanction of Years, perhaps of little besides; such is the Course of Victualling at Sea.

Histories of Medicine inform us, that many Remedies now ju— in the highest Esteem, were at their first Introduction deemed either of little or no Effect, or very pernicious; for Instance the Peruvian Bark, and Quick-Silver: It is not Impossible that the Hop Beer will meet the Same fa—

Further in favour of Hop Beer, it may not be unnecessary to o— that the Ingredients of which it is composed are the produce of this Country and of our West Indian Isles; and that if on Trial it answers t— purpose intended in the Essay, real advantages will accrue to the Hop a— Sugar Planter, and a considerable Increase to the Publick Revenue: Shou— this Scheme contribute to the preservation of the Health of our brave Seamen, Promote the Interest of the Hop and Sugar Planters and add to t— Publick Revenue, it is Humbly hoped the Author of it will be thought t— Merit Some share of favour.

FIG. 19 (OPPOSITE)
Essay on the means of preventing sea scurvy at sea, unknown author, about 1770, ADL/M/1/1

FIG. 20 (RIGHT)
Thos Trotter M.D. (Physician to the Grand Fleet), Daniel Orme, 1 May 1796, engraving, 174 × 119mm, PAD3448

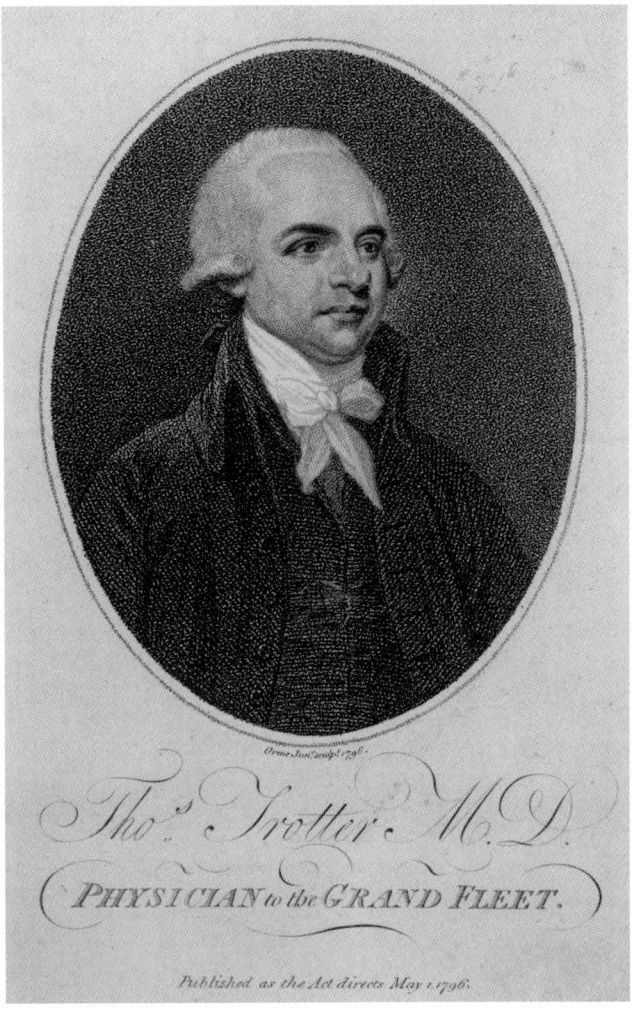

corn, alternately boiled; to which was added a sufficiency of Guinea pepper, and a small proportion of palm oil and common salt', would not protect them from the ravages of the disease. Trotter also pointed to the conditions below deck as disastrous for general health. Here, people were chained for 15 to 16 hours a day in intense heat, forced to lie on their sides 'and so close locked in one another's arms, that it is not possible to tread among them'. The first image of the conditions of enslaved people on board the ship *Brooks* was produced by William Elford and the Plymouth Society for Effecting the Abolition of the Slave Trade (SEAST) in late 1788. It was later amended by the London SEAST Committee and republished by their Quaker printer James Phillips, for distribution to MPs in 1789 (fig. 21).

Trotter noted that the symptoms, including gums 'separating in black masses from the teeth', 'pains and weaknesses in their extremities', 'ulcers', 'delirium' and 'haemorrhages from the nose', did not affect the crew in the same way. Already he put this down at least partially to a difference in diet, the crew having access to fresh vegetables which they purchased on land. By the time they reached Antigua, 40 enslaved African people had been buried at sea, and Trotter estimated that 300 were suffering from different degrees of scurvy. Disgusted by what he had seen, he left *Brooks*, returning to Edinburgh to continue his medical studies.

FIG. 21 *Plan and sections of a slave ship* 'Brooks', James Phillips, 1789, print on paper, 706 × 467mm, ZBA2745

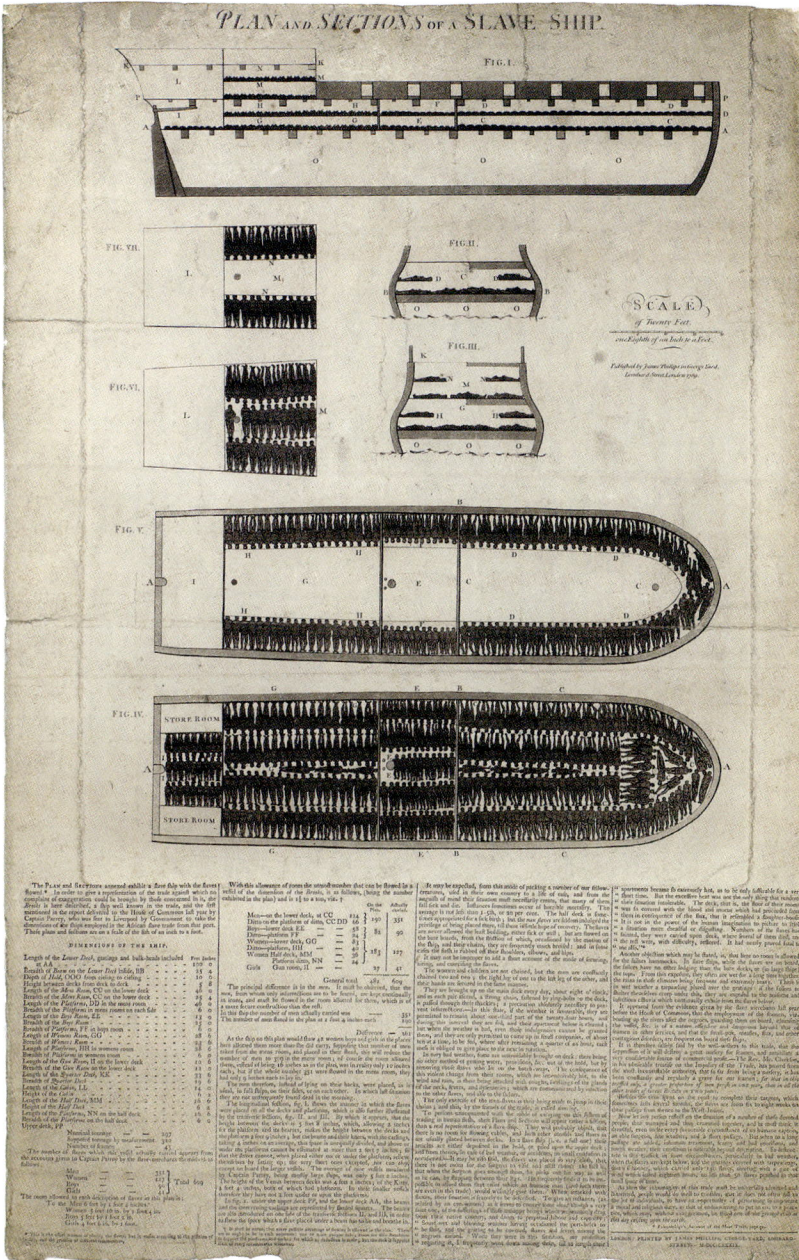

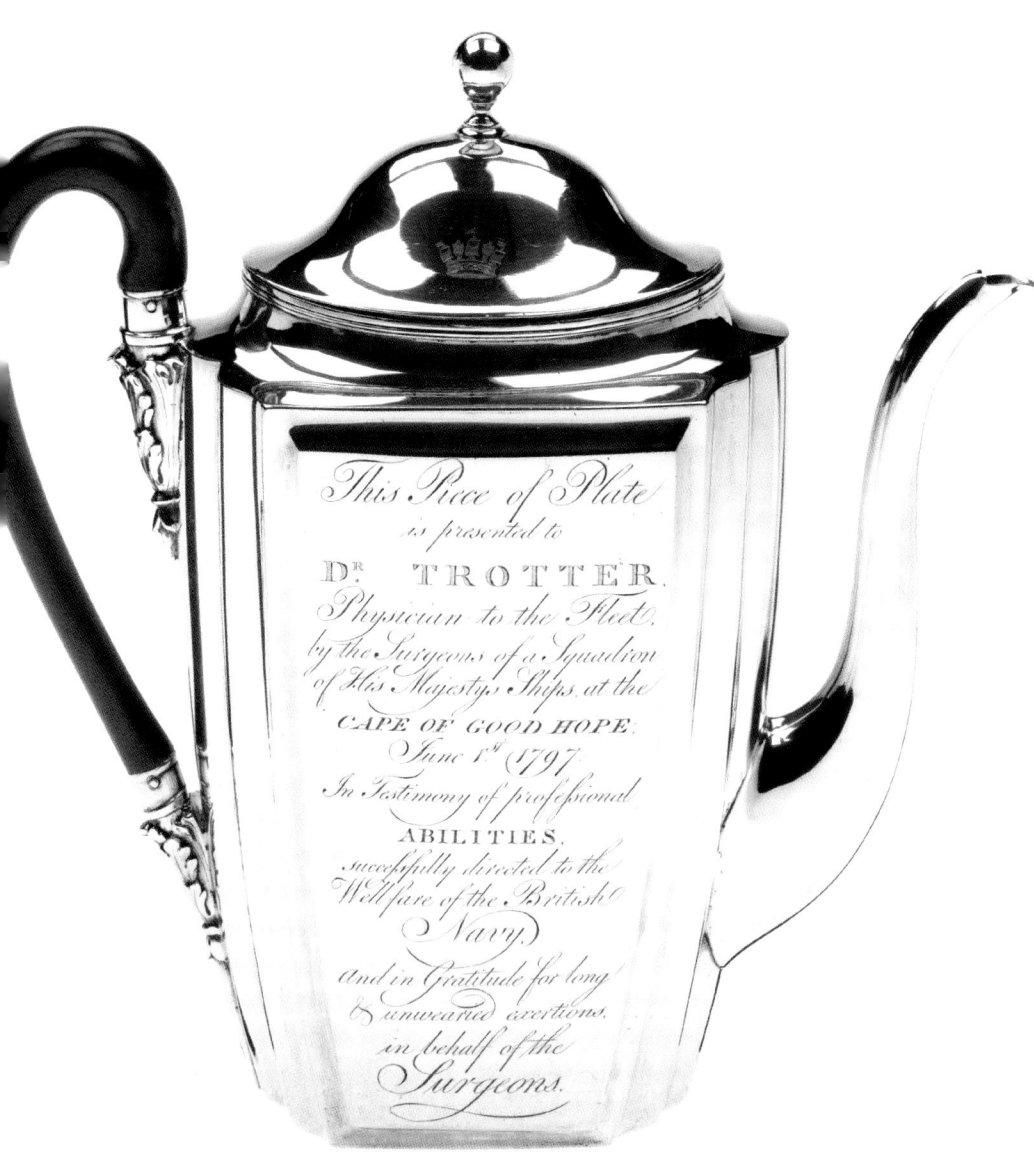

In 1786, his experiences led him to publish *Observations on the Scurvy*, with a second edition appearing in 1792. He theorised that scurvy was the result of a lack of oxygen, or 'vital air', in the affected tissues, arguing that it was the oxygen in acid fruits that restored the body to health. This helped explain why those at sea, and particularly those held in such dreadful conditions, were more vulnerable, since confined spaces below decks prevented the necessary oxygen entering the lungs through respiration. Nonetheless, as is always the case with this story, his embrace of citrus was not wholehearted and he expressed concern regarding the corrosive effect of too much citric acid, which he thought might damage the digestive system and prevent some of the benefits. Unlike some other theorists however, Trotter did not believe fruit acid could simply be replaced with an alternative, such as the sulphuric acid in oil of vitriol. Rather, he believed that different acids had different properties, which directly impacted their ability to oxygenate the body. When serving as physician to the Channel Fleet in 1795, Trotter ensured fresh food was provided, though he still believed in the use of citrus as a treatment rather than a preventative (fig. 22).

In 1781, less than a year after his appointment as physician to the West Indies Fleet, Gilbert Blane (1749–1834) issued a strongly worded 'memorial' to the Admiralty (fig. 23).

FIG. 22 Silver coffee pot presented to the naval physician Dr Thomas Trotter, Henry Chawner, about 1795, 280 × 250 × 105mm, PLT0186

By the Commissioners for
executing the Office of Lord
High Admiral of Great
Britain & Ireland &c.ᵃ

To Doctor Gilbert Blane

Whereas we have thought fit to
appoint you Physician to the Squadron
of His Majesty's Ships and Vessels
employed and to be employed at
Barbadoes, the Leeward Islands and
the Seas adjacent, You are hereby
authorized and required forthwith
to go on board the said Squadron
and take upon you the Charge of
Physician thereof accordingly,
and duly to execute the same,

He reported that of 1,600 deaths out of around 120,000 men, only 60 were the result of enemy action. This meant that the remaining 1,540 had died of other causes, the majority falling to infectious diseases but many others to scurvy. His resultant proposal that the fleet be supplied with fresh fruits and vegetables failed to influence the Admiralty. Blane was not alone in finding his advice ignored. In 1785, an East India Company surgeon wrote to the Admiralty about his experience in the treatment of scurvy. Over the course of six voyages to India, he had found that lemon and lime juice preserved in brandy provided an effective cure. He considered it his duty to inform them. Sadly, the Admiralty responded that rob of lemons and oranges had already been tried on many occasions and found to be of no value. They remained committed to portable soup, wort, sauerkraut and other such foods now known to be useless.

But this was not the end of the tale, nor of Gilbert Blane's role in the fight against scurvy. On returning to London in 1783, Blane was appointed to St Thomas' Hospital and soon became physician to the Royal Household. He published two editions of a treatise titled *Observations on the Diseases incident to Seamen* (1785, 1789) which upheld some traditional ideas such as the value of sauerkraut and sugar but argued that lemons and oranges were the most effective treatment. He believed particularly in the efficacy of juice rather than the rob, which he correctly intuited

FIG. 23 Detail of Admiralty order appointing Gilbert Blane as physician, 2 Oct 1781, BLA/58

was made less effective by heating. When Admiral Gardner (1742–1808/9) prepared to sail to India on *Suffolk* in 1793, Blane advised him to ask the Admiralty for a supply of lemon juice. This led to another important experiment, which once again proved the importance of citrus in the fight against scurvy. The men were given two-thirds of a liquid ounce every day and by the time they arrived in Chennai (then Madras) after 23 weeks, they had not lost a single man to the disease. Where scurvy had raised its head, an increased dose of juice had provided a cure.

The success of the experiment was followed in 1795 with Blane's appointment as a commissioner of the Board of Sick and Wounded Sailors, formerly the Sick and Hurt Board, where he had enough influence to persuade the Admiralty to issue lemon juice to naval ships. It is worth remembering that the terms lemon juice and lime juice were used interchangeably at this time so we cannot say for certain exactly which juice was received. Either way, by the time of the Battle of Trafalgar in 1805, scurvy was largely eliminated as a major issue in the Royal Navy. Over that 20-year period, naval ships were issued with approximately 1.5 million gallons of juice. It was not until 1854 that the Shipping Act obliged owners of merchant ships to make the same allotment. Even so, many owners purchased tainted juice at a lower cost or simply continued not to supply any at all. The Act became stricter in 1867.

Empirical evidence, rather than medical theory, had long demonstrated that scurvy could be cured, and even prevented, by citrus fruits and other fresh fruits and vegetables, even if the reasons for this remained unclear. While it might seem that this simple truth had at last been accepted, there was a final twist in the tale, threatening this hard-won conclusion.

The Victorian era saw great interest in polar exploration, both to the Arctic and the Antarctic. There was a scientific rationale for this but also a commercial one, as ships sought out the elusive North-West Passage to trading centres in Asia. By the latter part of the nineteenth century, the Navy was confident that, with correct provisioning of lime juice, its crews could survive at least two years in the Polar regions without contracting scurvy. So when the disease broke out among the crew of an 1875 Arctic expedition, affecting 60 men and killing three in only a year, there was a parliamentary inquiry. Ultimately, the expedition leader Captain George Nares (about 1831–1915) was held to be responsible, on the basis that he had failed to provide lime juice to the sledging parties. There was instant opposition to the verdict against Nares, including those who pointed out that lime juice was not generally taken on sledging expeditions, since it would simply freeze and could not be defrosted during nightly stops. Others brought up instances of scurvy breaking out on ships where crews did have access to lime juice. Indeed, one man found his scurvy returning even after it was administered. The case for citrus was once again called into doubt. At the end of the century the Royal Society authorised a committee to consider scurvy in light of new medical theories that showed many diseases were in fact caused by microscopic organisms. This 'germ theory' of disease still holds today, as we understand many illnesses to be the result of microorganisms such as bacteria or viruses. The results undermined centuries of progress in understanding the disease. The committee reported that scurvy was not after all a disease of deficiency but rather the result of bacteria, which grew on tainted food, specifically the meat carried on expeditions such as that led by Nares (figs 24 and 25). At least one naval surgeon now proposed that lime juice was beneficial only insofar as it provided an antibacterial mouthwash.

This hypothesis also explained why a diet of fresh meat seemed to prevent outbreaks of scurvy in the Arctic. Already from the early 1850s, small, private expeditions had recognised that the Inuit diet contained large amounts of fresh or very lightly cooked meat but little fruit or vegetables (fig. 26). Yet scurvy

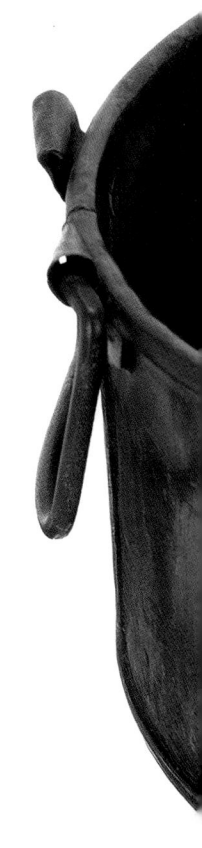

FIG. 24 A metal stew pan made for the British Arctic Expedition led by Captain George Nares, 1875, copper, 152 × 248mm, AAA4006

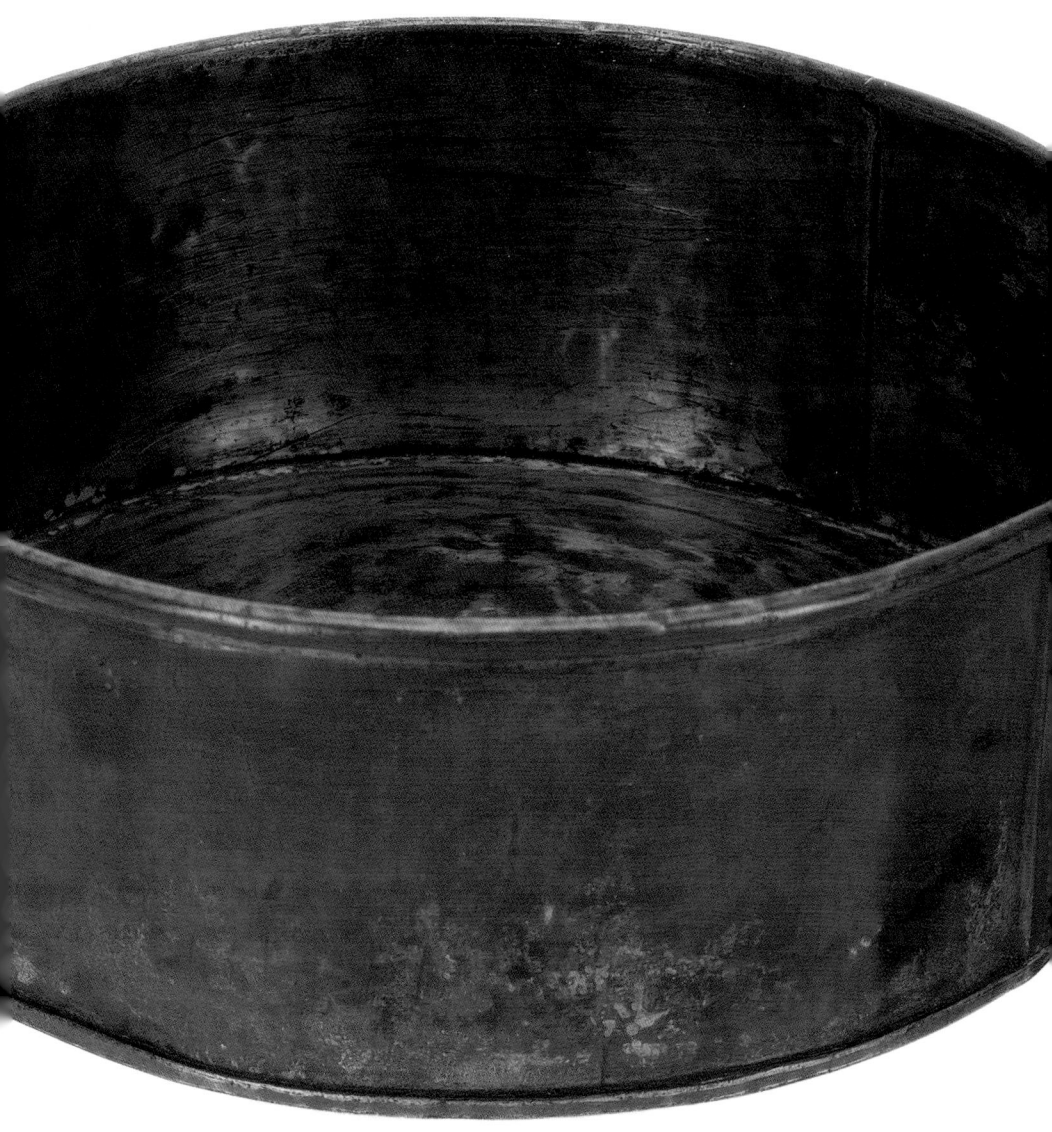

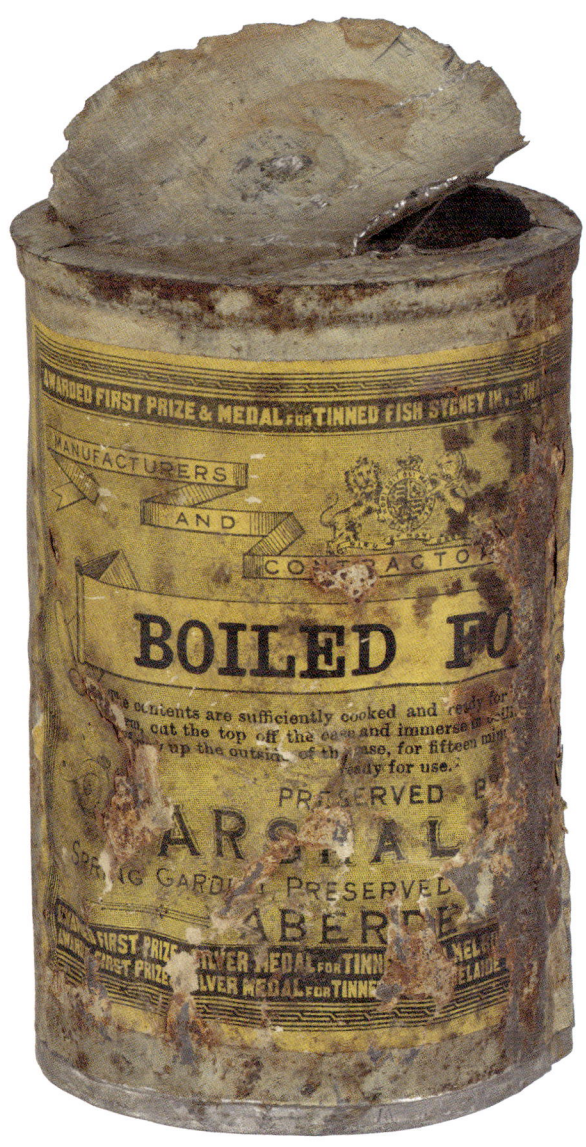

was not a common problem. An Admiralty committee of 1877 recommended that crews in polar regions consume fresh meat as often as possible and the Royal Society also promoted it as an antiscorbutic. Theories as to why this should be the case included that lactic acid in the muscles of animals had a similar effect to citric acid in lemons, limes and oranges. With the new proposition, which argued scurvy was the result of contaminated tins of meat, the value of fresh game was simply that it replaced the need to eat tinned meat in the first place (fig. 25). The truth of the matter is very different. Since most animals manufacture their own vitamin C, it is spread throughout their tissues. As such, consuming fresh meat that is raw or lightly heated provides a reasonable source of ascorbic acid.

With hindsight, it is difficult to understand how centuries of evidence could be so easily cast aside in favour of a theory that was simply wrong. Nor was it the only hypothesis to go against the lessons of fresh vegetables and citrus, which had seemed well and truly learned mere decades earlier. By 1907, the respected medical textbook *Modern Medicine: Its Theory and Practice* laid out several other contemporary ideas. These included the notion that scurvy was the result of deficiency of potassium in the blood, that it was caused by 'acid intoxication' or a reduction in alkalinity of the blood, or 'the

FIG. 25 Tinned meat, originally containing boiled fowl, manufactured by Marshall & Co for the Royal Navy, 1888–90, steel and paper, 135 × 80mm, AAB0009

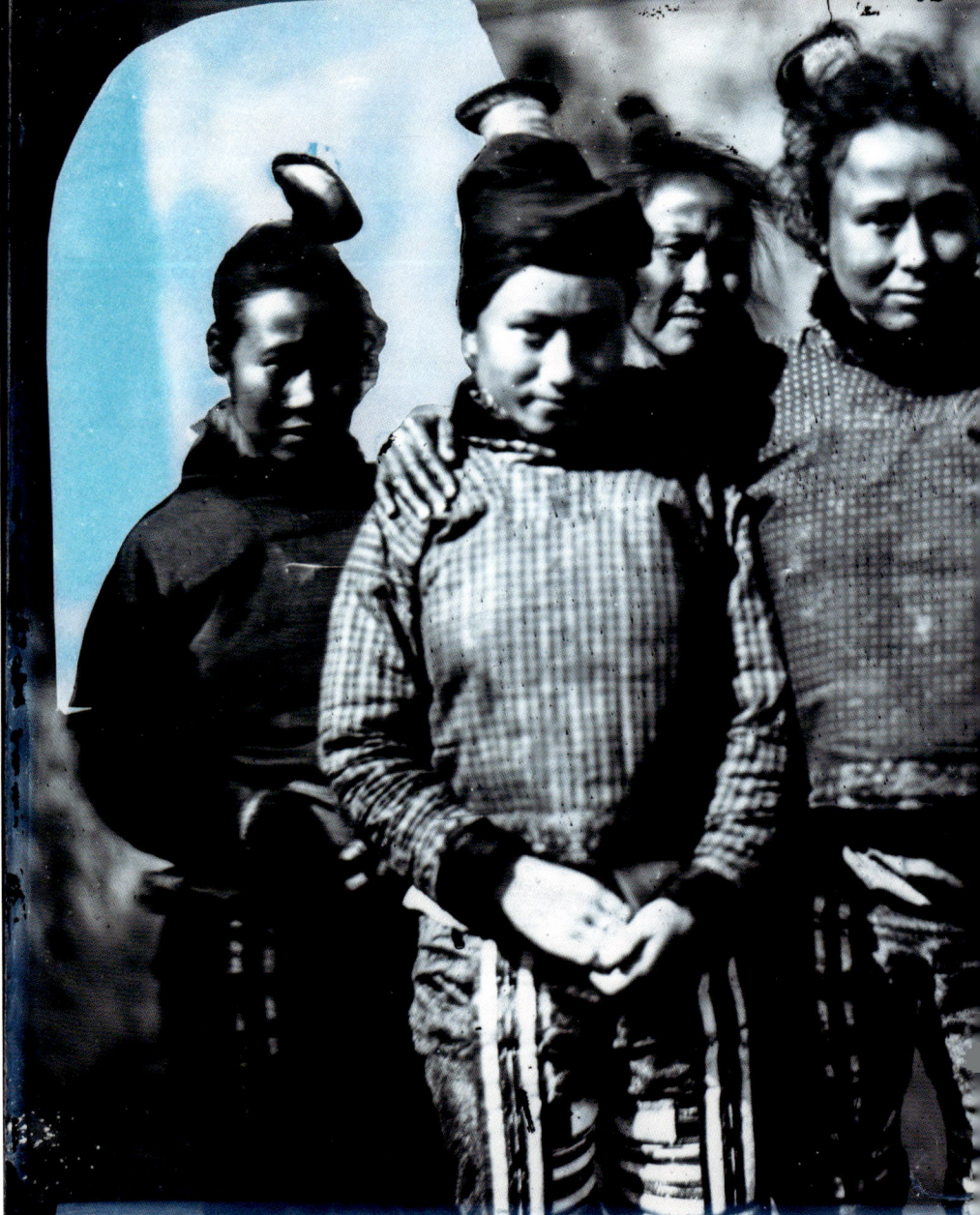

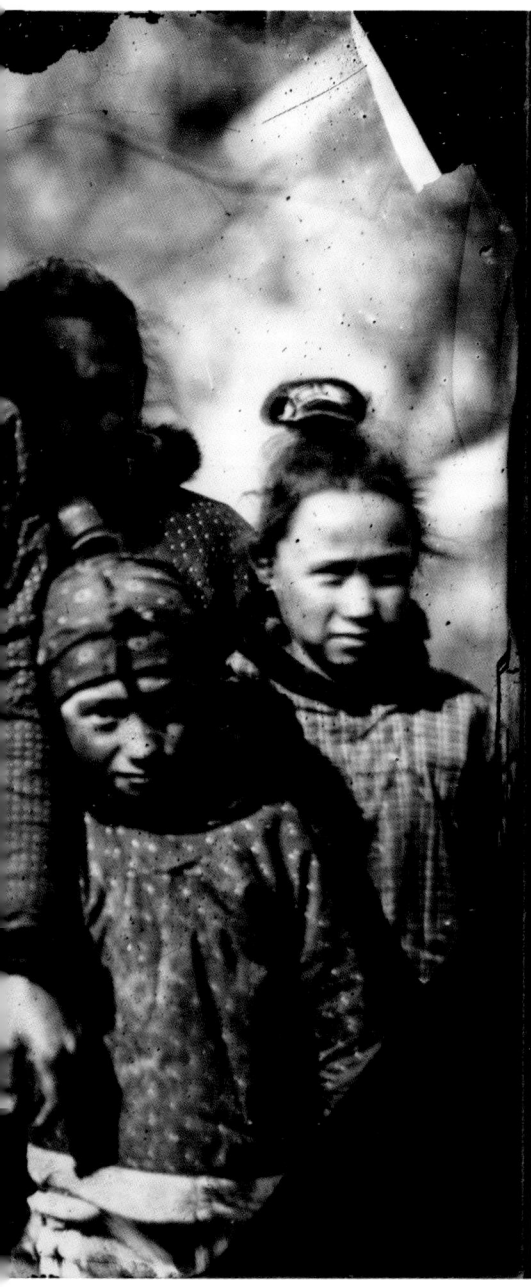

FIG. 26
Seven Inuit girls and women from West Greenland, Captain Edward Augustus Inglefield, 1854, wet collodion negative, 162 × 212mm, G4262

view which has been recently gaining ground', that 'scurvy is the result of a specific infection which takes place through the mouth'. The textbook sums up its account by proposing that while a 'deficiency of fresh vegetables' plays a part in the disease, it is not the whole story. It also argues that 'overwork', exposure to cold, damp climates and insanitary conditions lowered resistance and allowed the illness to take hold.

Though it seems wrongheaded to the modern reader, it is important to stress the complexity of the situation. Simply put, lime juice often failed to prevent scurvy, even though it continued to be compulsory on British ships. The reasons for this are themselves complicated and, in many cases, hard to define. In the first instance, from the 1790s to the 1850s research suggests that the quantities of juice carried on ship were not enough to ensure a daily ration for all those on board. Then, from the 1860s, the Admiralty switched from the Sicilian lemon to the West Indian lime in its production of juice for the Navy. It was discovered in experiments in the early 1900s that lime juice contained roughly two-thirds the concentration of vitamin C of lemons, and there is reason to believe that aspects of the production process of commercial lime juice further reduced the quantities of ascorbic acid. Possibly the concentration of vitamin C was affected by the long periods the juice spent in settling tanks. Alternatively, it may have been pumped through copper tubing; copper is now known to have a destructive effect on vitamin C. It is also likely that there was simply considerable variance in the efficacy of different supplies. Add to this the interchangeability of the terms 'lemon' and 'lime' juice over the entire period and it is even harder to form a concrete picture. What is clear is that the value of citrus in both preventing and curing scurvy remained vulnerable to challenge even into the 1900s.

Chapter 4
The Discovery of Vitamin C

As shown, in the early 1900s the confusion over the causes and treatment of scurvy remained alive and well. Where at one point it seemed that citrus had been accepted as the cure, new theories called this into question. While many believed that poor diet may provide the foundation for the illness, by weakening resistance, some still thought there was some external factor, some infectious agent that ultimately caused the disease. But things were about to change.

Two Norwegian scientists, Alex Holst (1860–1931, fig. 27), Professor of Hygiene and Bacteriology at the University of Christiana and Theodor Frølich (1870–1947, fig. 28), a paediatrician with a particular interest in infantile scurvy, were to play an important part. Holst was researching beriberi, a disease which we now know is caused by a deficiency of thiamine (vitamin B1). For his studies, which would look at the preventative merits of different substances, he made a hugely fortunate choice in his selection of animal model. Eschewing the chickens that had previously been used for this research, and also dogs which were often used in French and German feeding trials, he instead opted for the guinea pig. As we have seen, guinea pigs are one of the few species, like humans, that do not synthesise their own vitamin C, though of course Holst did not know this. When these animals began to show symptoms of scurvy during the trial, he brought Frølich on board and they were able to conclude that the scurvy present in the guinea pigs was identical to that seen in human beings. They had also revealed that scurvy could be caused by diet alone. Their experiments came to an end in 1913 but laid the groundwork, and provided the perfect animal model, for future studies in this area.

Fortunately for this story, interest in diet and nutrition was gripping members of the scientific community. In 1912, Frederick

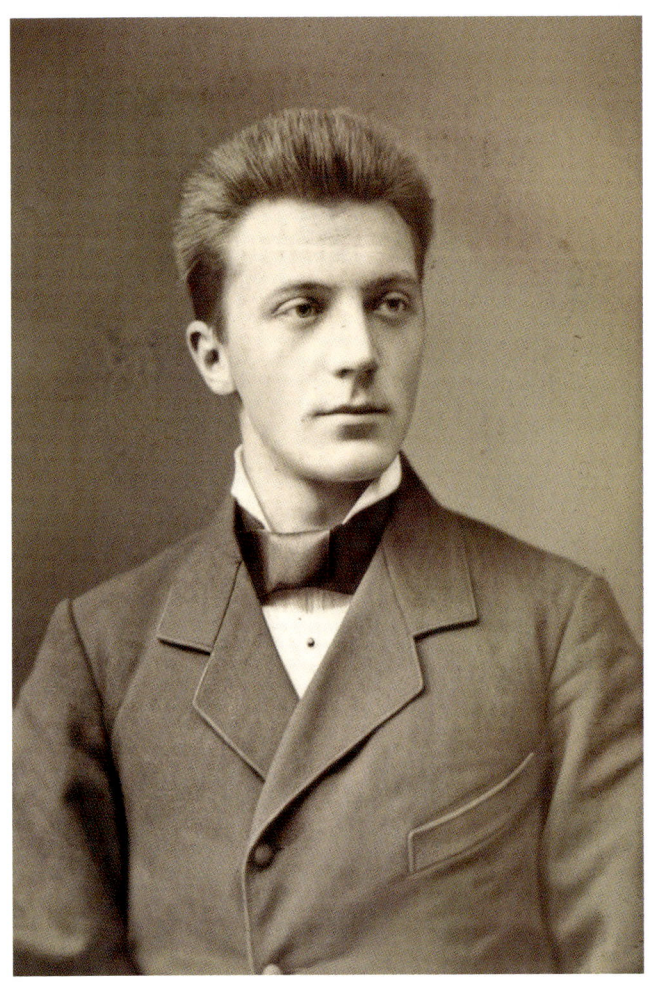

FIG. 27 (ABOVE) *Axel Holst*, Frederick Klem, 1880, Oslo Museum

FIG. 28 (OPPOSITE) *Theodor Frølich*, unknown photographer, about 1910, University of Kristiania, Oslo

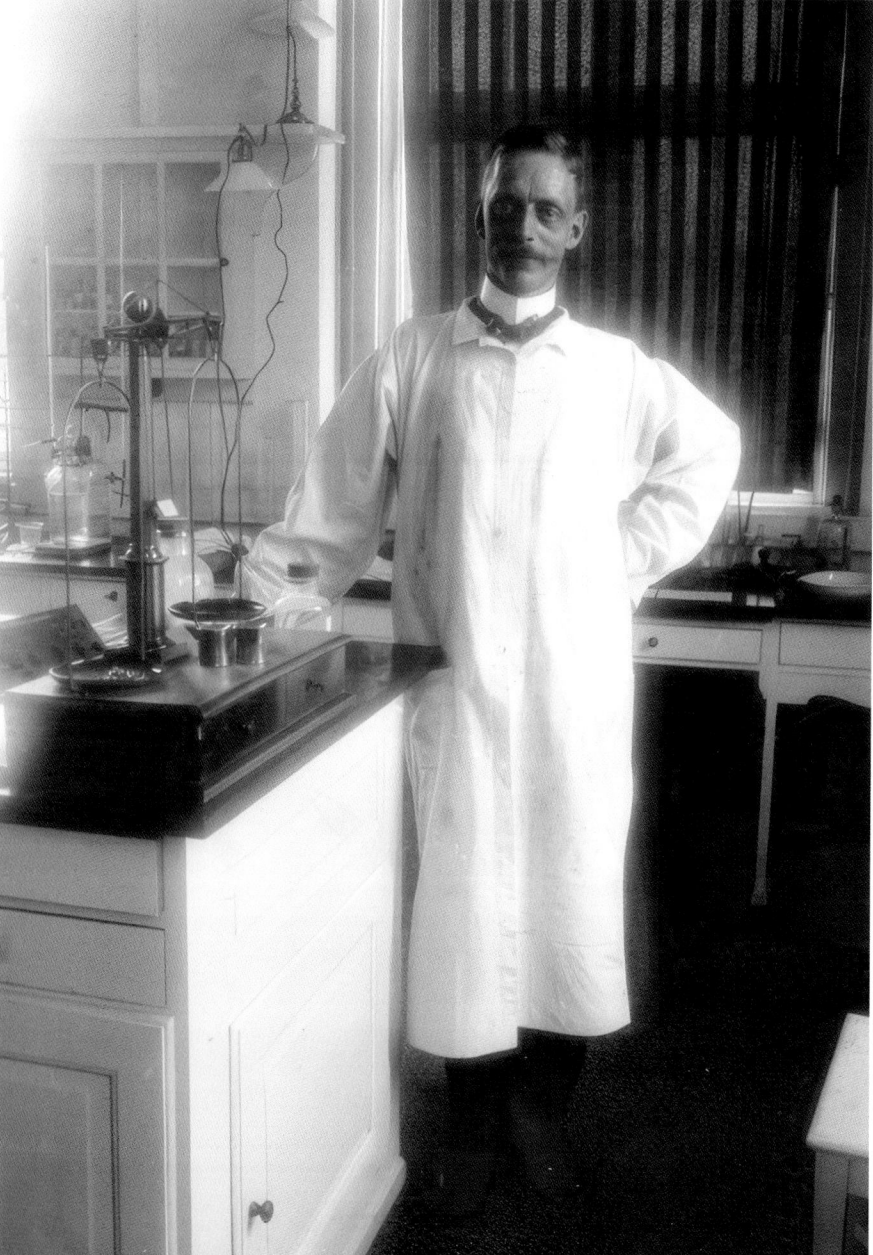

Gowland Hopkins's (1861–1947) experiments with rats led to arguments that a complete diet required small amounts of certain distinct compounds. That same year, Casmir Funk (1884–1967), a young Polish chemist working at the Lister Institute in London, proposed that four diseases including scurvy, beriberi, rickets and pellagra were caused by dietary deficiency of specific factors, which he termed 'vitamines'. Though some of the detail of his work was later disproved, the name 'vitamine', later changed to 'vitamin', provided a useful point of focus. Then, in 1913, American scientists revealed that certain fats contained a substance essential to growth in rats. Following the publication of a paper outlining their research, Elmer McCollum (1879–1967) and Marguerite Davis (1887–1967) were credited with discovering the first 'vitamin'. They had called the substance 'fat-soluble factor A', though it later came to be known as vitamin A.

There were, however, setbacks soon after; the story of scurvy had never been straightforward. A paper from McCollum's laboratory in 1917 concluded that scurvy was not in fact a deficiency disease. In part, this verdict was based on inconsistencies in experiments with guinea pigs where, given the same diet, some contracted scurvy and others did not. This was then added to the fact that rats did not develop scurvy under conditions in which it emerged in both human beings and guinea pigs. This presented two options: either guinea pigs and humans required something in their diet that rats did not, or scurvy was not a deficiency disease in the obvious sense. The latter seemed likely, since all the species were highly developed mammals and should therefore possess the same dietary needs.

Meanwhile, back in London, a group at the Lister Institute, led by biochemist Harriette Chick (1875–1977) (fig. 29), were still looking into scurvy and pellagra as diseases borne of dietary deficiency. In 1916, Chick was tasked with carrying out feeding trials after cases of both illnesses appeared in soldiers serving in the Middle East. The hope was that the group at the Lister Institute could advise on what foods should be added to army rations to ensure all nutritional needs were met. The team was almost entirely comprised of women, since their male colleagues were required for the war effort. Through their experiments they demonstrated that it was a question of quantity, as well as the type, of food that determined whether a guinea pig was likely to develop scurvy. This was not a factor that had been considered before, with differences in consumption by individual animals being overlooked, and so explained some of the variances in previous experiments.

Despite some continuing uncertainty, scientists were now searching for the mystery factor, which seemed to prevent

FIG. 29
Harriette Chick, front row, second from right, from Lister Institute Group photograph, 1907, Wellcome Collection

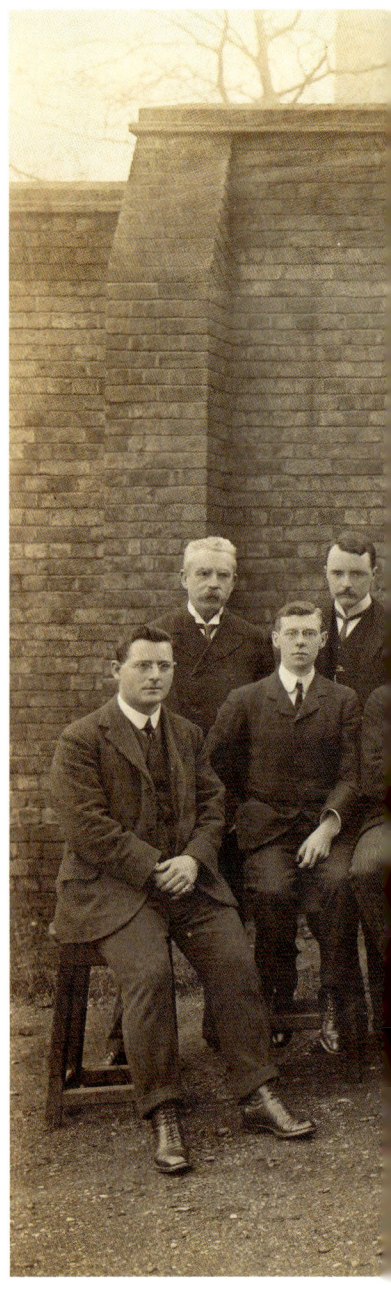

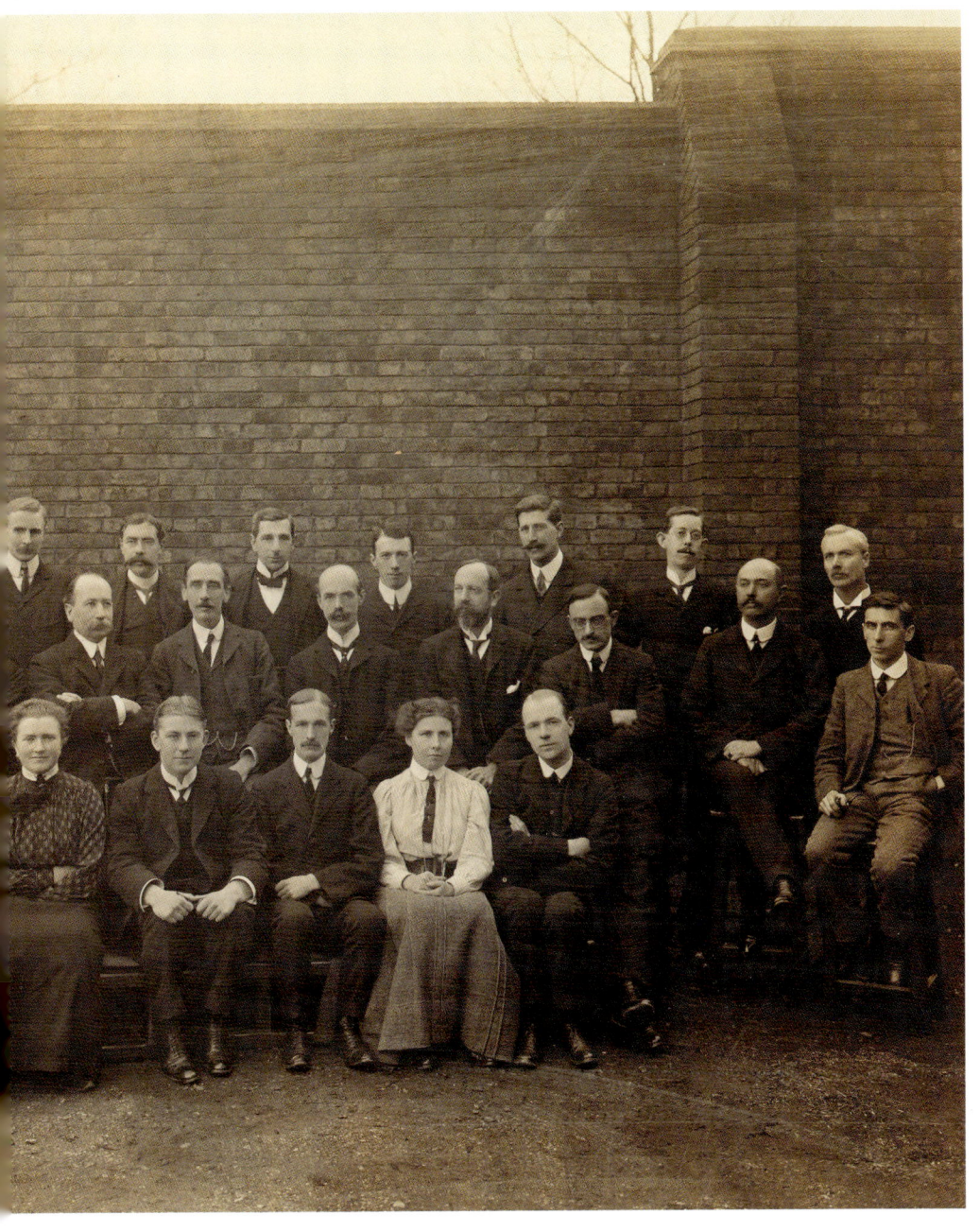

scurvy. As 'fat-soluble factor A' and also 'water-soluble factor B' had already been identified by McCollum's laboratory, those convinced that scurvy was a disease of deficiency were now seeking a factor 'C'.

Isolation of this factor was finally achieved by the Hungarian physiologist Albert Szent-Györgyi (1893–1986, fig. 30). Szent-Györgyi was investigating the chemical changes that result when cells make use of nutrients in food, such as proteins, fats and carbohydrates. In the process, he came to understand there was an as yet unknown substance involved which was present in both citrus fruit and the adrenal glands of animals. Szent-Györgyi went to work at the University of Cambridge in 1927 where he sought to isolate this substance and ultimately established its chemical formula. When writing up his findings in a paper, he initially wanted to call the molecule 'Ignose', a joke drawing on the words 'I don't know' and the suffix 'ose', which is used to indicate sugars. In the same vein, he also suggested calling it 'Godnose' but both were rejected by his editor. Instead, the substance came to be known as 'hexuronic acid' and Szent-Györgyi received his PhD for the discovery.

In 1930, Szent-Györgyi returned to Hungary, where he headed the Department of Medical Chemistry at the University of Szeged. While in post, he instructed American physician Joseph Svirbely to study the antiscorbutic properties of

FIG. 30 Albert Szent-Györgyi, unknown photographer, about 1930, University of Cambridge

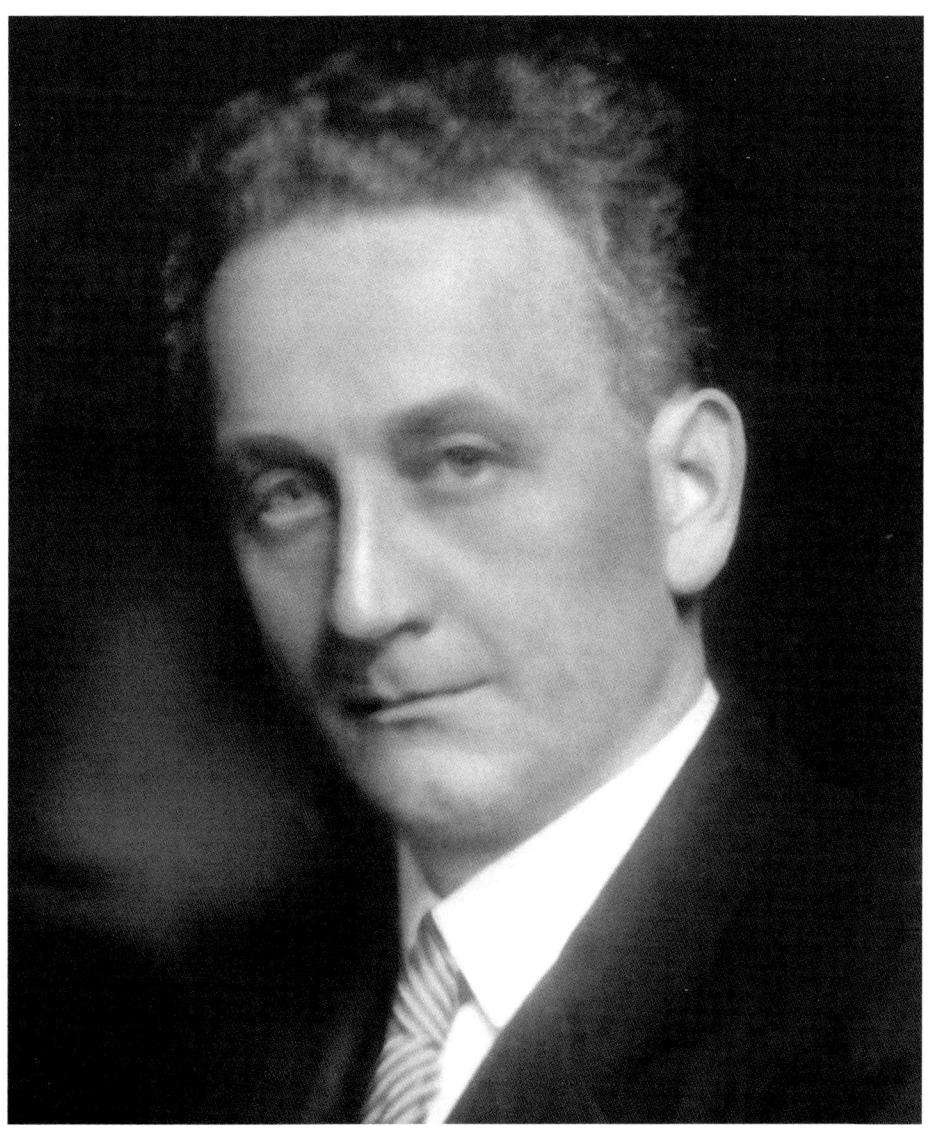

hexuronic acid. Svirbely had previously worked with Charles Glen King (1896–1988) at Pittsburgh on research into vitamin C. Glen King had also been striving to isolate the vitamin from lemon juice and in 1932 published a paper with W.A. Waugh reporting that they had managed to obtain a substance that corresponded to Szent-Györgyi's hexuronic acid. They found that this substance prevented scurvy in guinea pigs during nutritional trials. Two weeks later, Szent-Györgyi and Svirbely published their own paper, which offered the same conclusion. Vitamin C had, at last, been discovered, though the question of who deserved credit created a level of resentment between the American and Hungarian scientific communities. In the end, Szent-Györgyi was to receive the Nobel Prize for Physiology and Medicine in 1937 for a full body of work but with particular reference to vitamin C.

Further experiments were conducted to determine the extent to which scurvy, as it appeared in humans, could be explained purely by a deficiency of ascorbic acid. In 1939 Jon Crandon, a surgeon affiliated with Harvard Medical School, put himself on a limited diet which excluded vitamin C. After 12 weeks, he became fatigued and by 19, he began to experience physical symptoms including dry, rough skin and hard lumps at the base of the hairs on his legs. After continuing on the diet, small haemorrhages broke out on his lower legs and a wound deliberately inflicted 26 weeks in had not healed at all after 10 days. A similar experiment was carried out with conscientious objectors in Sheffield during the Second World War. After 30 weeks without vitamin C, gums became swollen and spongy and began to bleed. After 36 weeks, one member of the group suffered cardiac symptoms following physical exercise, thought to be the result of a 'scorbutic haemorrhage'.

Efforts were soon made to determine the daily dietary requirements of vitamin C and in time, it was even possible to produce it synthetically. Vitamin pills were increasingly used in the Second World War and post-war period while food manufacturers began to fortify their products with essential vitamins.

Modern science was finally able to prove that the disease which so decimated ships' crews over the centuries was the result of a severe deficiency in vitamin C. The shipboard diet: biscuit, salt meat, cheese, pease and so on, provided effectively no ascorbic acid and made suffering, and in many instances death, inevitable. Countless physicians, surgeons, seafarers and admiralty officials, over hundreds of years, had poured their energies into finding a cause and cure for the illness. What is hard to understand in hindsight only, is that it took them so long. But without knowledge of vitamin C or of vitamins in general, with occupational hierarchies prioritising land-based physicians over shipboard surgeons, and with the need for economies alongside professional biases and even contradictory evidence, the time taken makes a lot more sense. Even the issuing of lime juice, as represented by the bottle with which this book began, was not foolproof, for reasons that simply could not be understood at the time. The long duration matters because of the number of lives impacted by the disease. That an answer came in the end is testament to the determination of many individuals whose commitment, imagination and curiosity eventually came to fruition.

FIG. 31 Lime juice bottle, late eighteenth century, glass, 268mm, ZBA7971

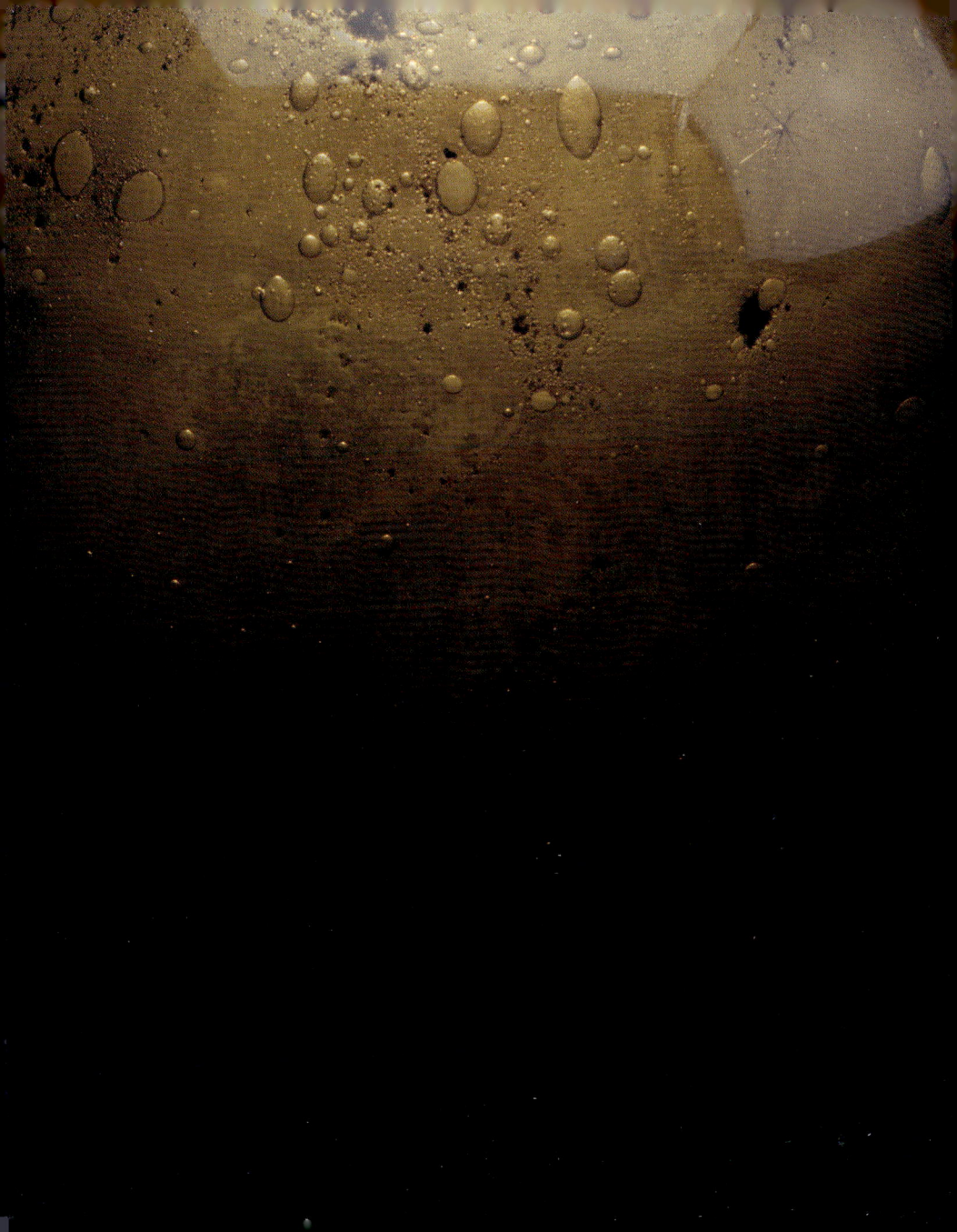

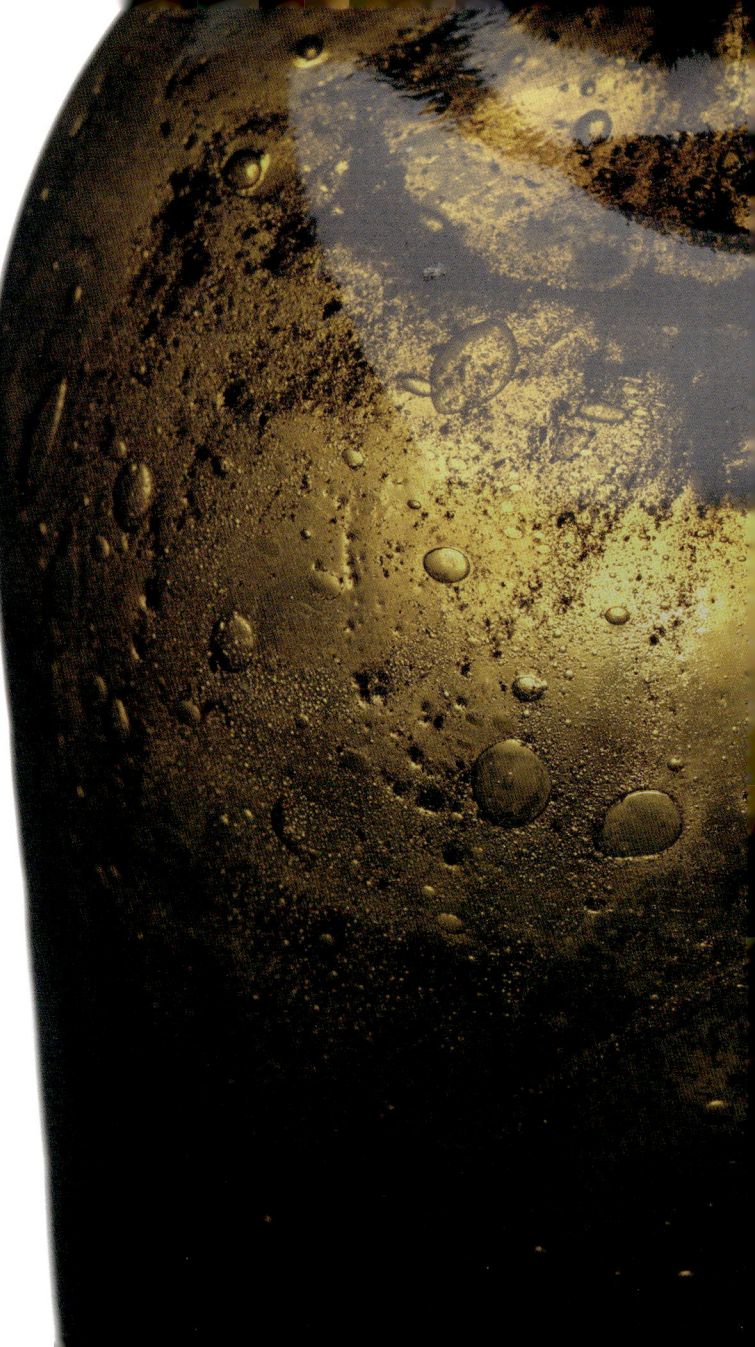

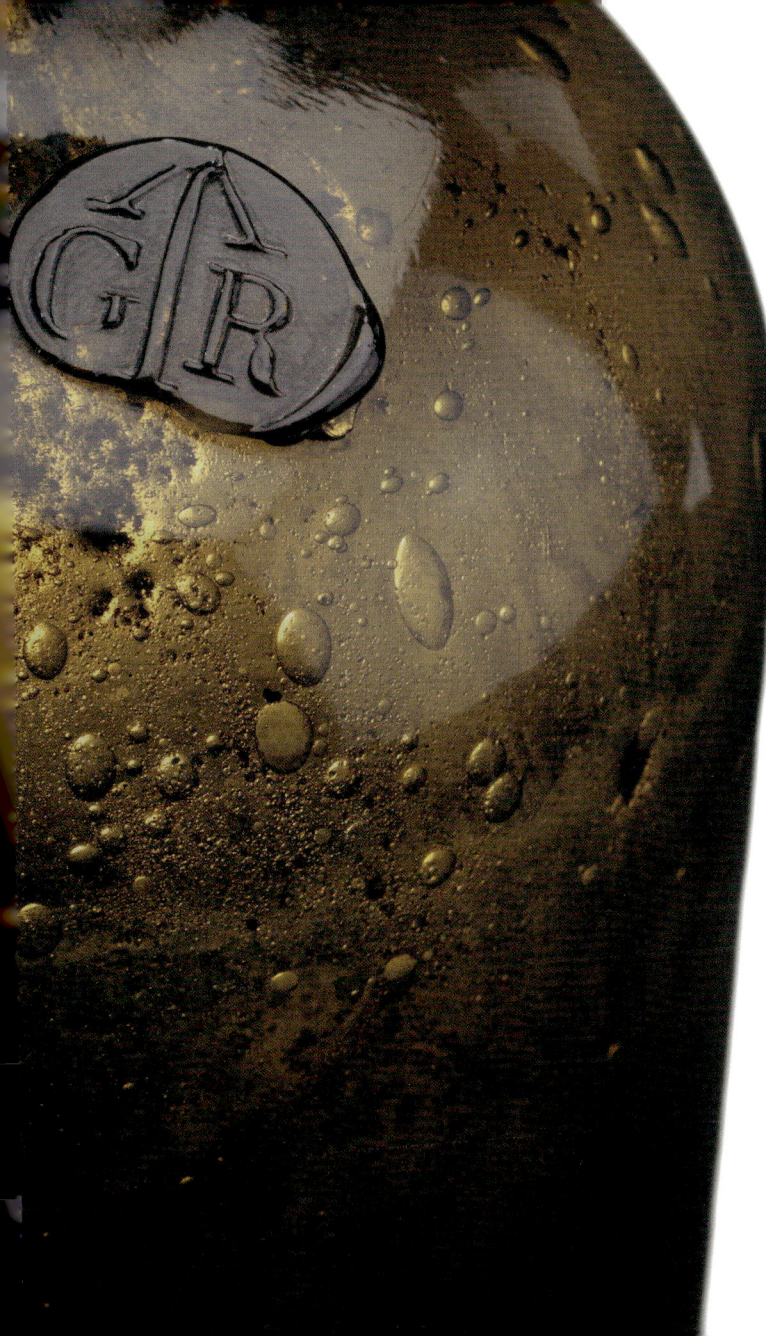

Further Reading

Carpenter, K.J., *The History of Scurvy and Vitamin C*, Cambridge University Press, Cambridge, 1986

Lamb, J., *Scurvy The Disease of Discovery*, Princeton University Press, Princeton, 2018

Williams, G., *The Prize of All the Oceans: The Triumph and Tragedy of Anson's Voyage Round the World*, HarperCollins, London, 1999

Bown, S.R., *Scurvy: How a Surgeon, a Mariner and a Gentleman Solved the Greatest Medical Mystery of the Age of Sail*, The History Press, Cheltenham, 2021

Macdonald, J.W., *Feeding Nelson's Navy: The True Story of Food at Sea in the Georgian Era*, Frontline Books, Barnsley, 2014

Kiple, K.F., et al., *The Cambridge World History of Human Disease*, Cambridge University Press, Cambridge, 1993

Acknowledgements

I am grateful for the assistance and support I received while writing this book. I would like to thank Susan Winchell-Sweeney and Dr Gwendolyn Saul of the New York State Museum for their assistance in finding an appropriate image relating to the Cartier voyage. I would also like to thank Darren Bonaparte, Director of the Tribal Historic Preservation Office for the Saint Regis Mohawk Tribe, for granting permission for the reproduction of this image (fig. 6).

A further debt of thanks is owed to colleagues at Royal Museums Greenwich including members of our Photo Studio who produced many of the images you see here. I would also like to express my sincere gratitude to the Publishing team, with whom I have worked closely since the book's inception and without whom it would simply not exist. Finally, I'd like to thank Dr Robert J. Blyth for his constant support throughout this project.

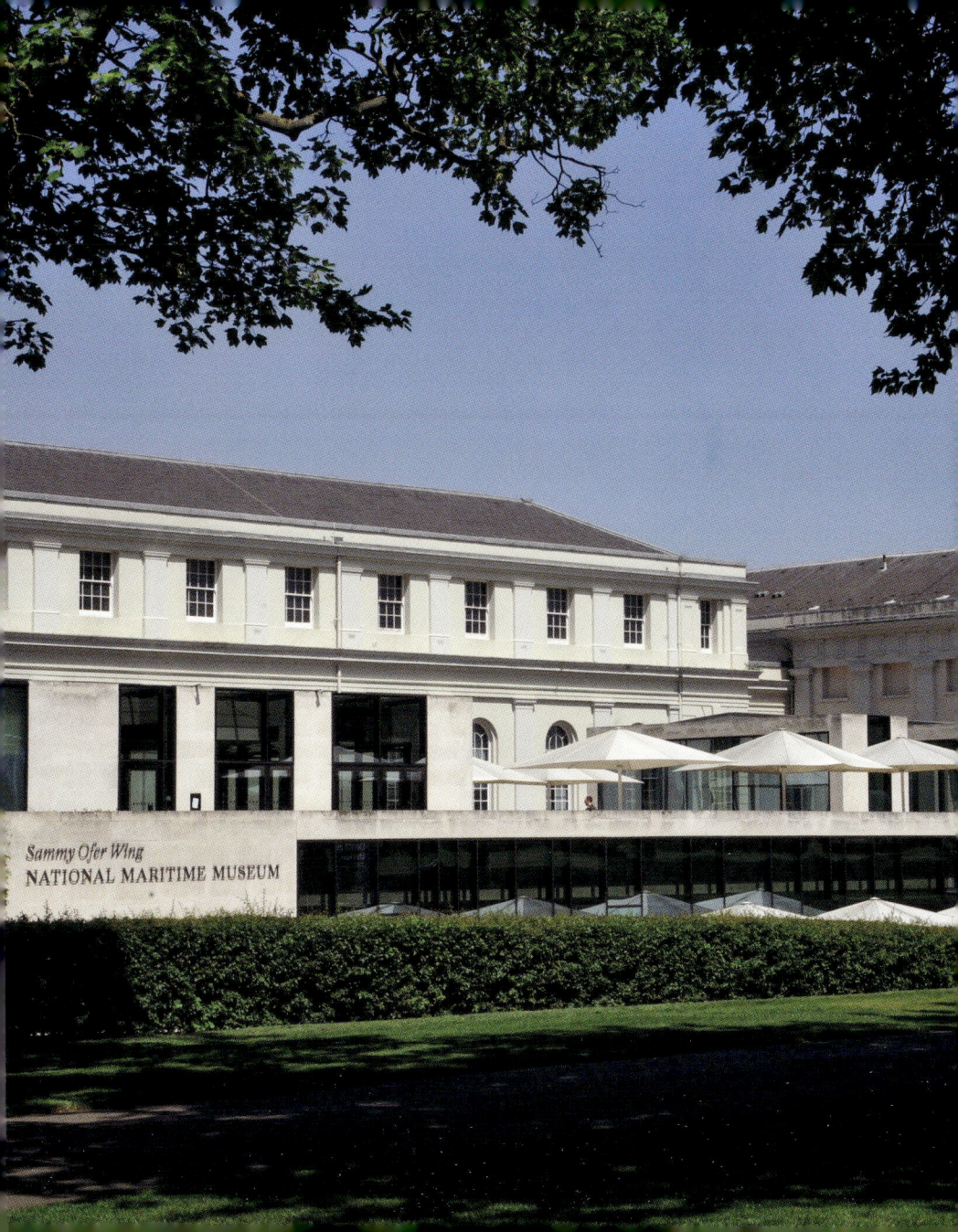

Picture Credits

Every attempt has been made to trace accurate ownership of copyrighted images in this book. Any errors or omissions will be corrected in subsequent editions provided notification is sent to the publisher. Unless otherwise stated, images are © National Maritime Museum, Greenwich, London.

pp. 12, 15 Courtesy Barts Health NHS Trust Archives
p. 19 Courtesy of the New York Museum with permission from the Saint Regis Mohawk Tribe
p. 26 © National Maritime Museum, Greenwich, London, Greenwich Hospital Collection
p. 30 © The National Archives, London
pp. 41, 80 Source: Wellcome Collection, London
p. 53 © Trustees of the British Museum

First published in 2025 by Royal Museums Greenwich
Park Row, Greenwich, London, SE10 9NF

publishing@rmg.co.uk

ISBN: 978-1-7391542-3-3

Text © National Maritime Museum, Greenwich, London
Lucy Dale has asserted her right under the Copyright, Designs and Patent Act 1988 to be identified as the author of this work.

At the heart of the UNESCO World Heritage Site of Maritime Greenwich are the four world-class attractions of Royal Museums Greenwich – the National Maritime Museum, the Royal Observatory, the Queen's House and *Cutty Sark*.

rmg.co.uk

All rights reserved. No part of this publication may be reproduced, stored in or introduced into a retrieval system, or transmitted in any form, or by any means (electronic, mechanical, photocopying, recording or otherwise) without the prior written permission of the publisher. Any person who commits any unauthorised act in relation to this publication may be liable to criminal prosecution and civil claims for damages. A CIP catalogue record for this book is available from the British Library.

Design by Peter Dawson, Ronja Rønning, www.gradedesign.com
Printed and bound by Green Leaf Production, Slovenia

10 9 8 7 6 5 4 3 2 1

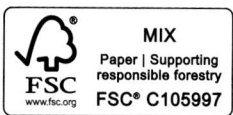